So You Qualified Abroad … The Handbook for Overseas Medical Graduates in GP Training

MANDY FRY

MB BS MPhil MRCGP
Portfolio GP and GP Educationalist

RICHARD MUMF~

PGCert Med Ed
Deputy GP Dean
Health Education Thames Valley

ANNELIESE GUERIN-LETENDRE

MA BEd (Hons) PgDip Management PgCert Coach
Professional Development Coach
Interpersonal Communications Specialist

Foreword by
ROGER NEIGHBOUR

DSc MA FRCGP FRCP
Past President, Royal College of General Practitioners

Radcliffe Publishing
London • New York

Radcliffe Publishing Ltd
St Mark's House
Shepherdess Walk
London N1 7BQ
United Kingdom

www.radcliffehealth.com

British Library Cataloguing in Publication Data

A catalogue record for this book is available from the British Library.

ISBN-13: 978 184619 998 1

The paper used for the text pages of this book is FSC® certified. FSC (The Forest Stewardship Council®) is an international network to promote responsible management of the world's forests.

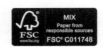

Typeset by Darkriver Design, Auckland, New Zealand
Manufacturing managed by 21 six

Contents

Foreword

Dr Roger Neighbour OBE DSc MA FRCGP FRCP
Past President, Royal College of General Practitioners
Author of *The Inner Consultation* and *The Inner Apprentice*

A few years ago I received an email inviting me to a conference on medical education to give a presentation about *'how GP trainees are taught and assessed in the United Kingdom'*. Easy, I thought, I know all about that. *'… in Toulouse, France'*, the email continued. Wonderful; France is a country I love, and here was an opportunity to visit a region whose scenery, food and wines are equally spectacular. *'… in French.'*

Ah. French is a language I'm reasonably fluent in, having learned it from the age of six at school in Scotland. Ask me to buy croissants in the patisserie, tell a waiter how I like my steak cooked, follow the news in a newspaper or even on television, and I'm fine. But explaining in a foreign language how the MRCGP curriculum was derived, or answering questions about the internal consistency of a multiple choice exam, would be a challenge of a different order. Still, I was willing to try. I could no doubt learn the specialist vocabulary, and the audience of French colleagues would surely be forgiving if I occasionally stumbled over the grammar and got the gender of a few nouns wrong.

'We would like you also to conduct some consultations with simulated patients for us to observe.' You mean, in French? *Naturellement.* No problem, I replied cheerfully, rashly, and ultimately embarrassingly. And so I learned the hard way that understanding colloquial and heavily accented French spoken in a merciless Gallic gabble, or trying to shepherd an uncomprehending patient through the red tape of a health system I myself had never experienced, is a world away from ordering the *plat du jour* on the *menu fixe*. On a conference platform my role-played efforts were amusing, possibly even endearing. No one actually came to harm. In real life, of course, I would have been a disaster. Lives – and this is no exaggeration – might have been lost.

In their introduction to this book, Mandy Fry and Richard Mumford offer you their congratulations on having embarked on a career path which, as they rightly observe, can bring you some of the greatest professional satisfaction to be found within medicine. You are indeed to be congratulated. Whether general practice was always your first career choice or something you have come to after a period of hospital specialisation; whether your ambition is to practise in the UK or to apply your hard-won skills to the benefit of other countries, other populations, you are joining a community of primary care doctors whose contribution to the world's health and happiness matters more and more. Like all systems of healthcare, Britain's National Health Service has its problems and its critics. But – be in no doubt – the UK's way of training and assessing the future general practitioner is second to none, and is admired around the globe.

Your colleagues in training whose lives, education and careers have taken place nowhere other than in Britain may indeed seem fortunate. Having experienced no other system, their knowledge of how the NHS operates is already deeply ingrained. Having spoken no other language, their command of English is already second nature. Having grown up in the British educational system, they already understand, even if they do not realise it, the conventions and nuances of British examinations. Not for them the potential for mutual misunderstanding that threatened my presentation in Toulouse and which on occasion may make some of your own consultations less effective than they might have been. That you find yourself at something of a disadvantage as you start your training for general practice is certainly no reflection on you. Neither is it the fault of 'the system' or 'the teaching' or 'the assessment process'. When cultures overlap, a degree of mutual awkwardness is inevitable. So as well as my congratulations you have my admiration and respect for your determination to overcome it.

But you deserve more. The differences in background, customs and experience which make GP training harder for some than for others cannot simply be shrugged off or legislated away. If they affect you, you deserve some proper help. Not the patronising kind of help that is prompted by pity or guilt. And not the kind of defensive help behind which political incorrectness tries to hide its face. You are entitled to the unconditional help one traveller extends to another simply because, though the journey is difficult, the destination is worth it.

This book offers exactly the right kind of help. The authors focus unflinchingly on those linguistic and cultural aspects of GP training and assessment where doctors who have trained mainly outside the UK can find themselves in difficulty. They rightly view the MRCGP examination not as an end itself but as a milestone on the way to a satisfying career. If you want to learn a few stock phrases and stereotypical behaviours that you hope will give your consultations the illusion of competence, then please look elsewhere. (Actually, please *don't* look elsewhere. Learn right now the lesson encapsulated in this book, namely, that becoming a good GP needs you to appreciate and cherish the unique complexities of every individual – patient and doctor alike.) The help you will find in these pages is practical without being over-simplified, comprehensive without being overwhelming. There are no quick fixes here, and nor should there be. Rather, the authors' approach will help you steadily develop the fluency, style and sensitivity that will best enable you to function as well as you deserve in British general practice.

Good luck!

Roger Neighbour
Bedmond, Hertfordshire
April 2014

About the authors

Dr Mandy Fry MB BS MPhil MRCGP
Mandy is a portfolio GP with a wide range of interests and has worked within postgraduate general practice education in Oxford for over 12 years. She gained her research degree looking at innovative approaches of using extensions to core GP training in a learner-centred way and has tried to maintain this perspective throughout her career in medical education. She particularly enjoys the challenge of working cross-culturally and has used this experience to develop a special interest in helping overseas medical graduates improve their communication skills. She is a native English speaker and has huge admiration for those who manage to routinely consult in a second language or in unfamiliar cultural situations. She is also an examiner for the MRCGP so she has a good understanding of the challenges involved in succeeding at assessments.

Richard Mumford PGCert Med Ed
Richard is the Deputy GP Dean at Health Education Thames Valley (HETV) and is also the Associate GP Dean with patch responsibility for Reading and Newbury. Richard has previously been a Programme Director in Banbury and has developed an interest in helping those struggling to get to grips with the consultation. He describes this as the most rewarding and interesting of his many roles. Richard is one of just a few Associate Deans who comes from a non-GP background. A potted career history is as a nurse in the 80s, a general manager in Leicester in the 90s, a Lecturer in Healthcare Management in the early 00s and has been involved in GP training in various roles since 2004. Richard also has an interest in GP foundation issues and is the lead for GP/ foundation issues for HETV. Richard designed and delivered one of the first ever CSA courses in early 2008. Richard is also an Honorary Associate Lecturer at De Montfort University and has an additional interest in quality management of training environments.

Anneliese Guerin-LeTendre MA BEd (Hons) PgDip Management PgCert Coach
Anneliese is a professional development coach, trainer and consultant, specialising in interpersonal and intercultural communication. Founder of Dialogue

Links, she brings an experience gained over 30 years of teaching, training and management in the public and private sector. The main focus of her work is accompanying individuals and teams as they resolve communications challenges at the interface between language and the many layers of culture – including professional, organisational and national.

Of Canadian and Irish origin, and a fluent French speaker, Anneliese's experiences of living in France and Canada have given her a personal and professional insight into the issues involved in cultural shift. An advocate of the 'co-active coaching' approach, she particularly values working alongside clients from a wide range of cultural backgrounds and promoting the exceptional advantages of culturally diverse teams and organisations.

Based in Health Education Thames Valley and Health Education Wessex, Anneliese works extensively in the National Health Service, coaching doctors across a wide range of specialisms and running regular workshops on culture, diversity and communication, including induction programmes for overseas medical graduates.

All three authors have been involved in running joint learning sets aimed particularly at individuals with issues around communication, many of whom are overseas medical graduates, within Health Education Thames Valley. These are affectionately referred to as Dragons' Den sessions, as the initial funding was achieved as part of a bid for educational innovation. We are not sure what this term conjures up for participants!

Acknowledgements

This book would not have happened without the inspiration of the overseas medical graduates who we have been privileged to work with in our monthly learning sets, so we would like to acknowledge them formally. We are particularly grateful to those who have been generous enough to share some of their personal stories, which you will find peppered throughout the book.

Introduction: setting the scene

Congratulations!

That might seem like a strange way to start a book, but we think there are several reasons why you deserve to be congratulated. We have aimed this book primarily at individuals who have qualified overseas and who have then decided to train to become general practitioners (GPs) in the United Kingdom (UK). However, it will also be relevant to those who are contemplating starting GP training and those who have just completed such training. Overseas medical graduates (OMGs) from other specialties and educationalists working with these individuals may also find it helpful.

At this stage it is worth pointing out that we use the phrase 'overseas medical graduates', or OMGs, throughout this book as meaning individuals whose primary medical qualification is from somewhere other than the UK. This phrase seems to have replaced the term 'international medical graduates', which some of you may be more familiar with. We can only apologise for the fact that its three-letter acronym OMG is used by some folk as text speak for Oh My God! We did not coin either phrase ...*

So back to the reasons why we think you should be congratulated.

1. By deciding to become a GP in the UK you have chosen one of the best jobs in the world, and one that we believe will give you more than adequate financial remuneration, as well as amazing job satisfaction for the rest of your life.

2. You may well have already achieved the first step – that of becoming a GP in the UK. This is no mean feat, as getting selected for general practice training is a competitive process.

3. Your decision to buy this book suggests you have recognised that your needs may be different from those who have qualified in the UK.

These three things are worth holding onto as you progress through this book and through your GP training. This is because there is significant evidence

---

Phrase notes
* 'to coin a phrase' – to create a new expression that is worthy of being remembered and repeated

that you may well find some aspects of your training more difficult than your UK colleagues, unfortunately. For example, for first attempts at the Clinical Skills Assessment (CSA) between 2010 and 2012, those from black and ethnic minority groups who qualified overseas were 15 times more likely to fail than white UK graduates (failure rate is 65%, compared with 4.5%).[1] Indeed, even getting selected for GP training is more of a challenge for those who qualified overseas.[2] If you have not heard those statistics before, they can be shocking. Indeed, one individual I know who travelled to the exam with three fellow OMGs suddenly realised that it was likely that only two of them would be successful at passing the exam at that attempt. Why this discrepancy exists is something that the Royal College of General Practitioners (RCGP), academics and OMGs themselves are all looking into[1,3-8] and the current debate about this is fascinating to follow. It is interesting, however, that it is similarly displayed across other postgraduate medical exams for other specialties.[9,10] As a counterbalance to these statistics, it is worth noting that in 2012 a quarter of the UK general practice workforce was made up of people who qualified overseas,[11] although admittedly many of them will have become GPs prior to the advent of the Membership of the Royal College of General Practitioners (MRCGP) exam becoming a prerequisite to practice.

With regard to the exam statistics, individuals with different perspectives inevitably have differing views as to why this might be the case. However, they can be broadly divided into three types of difference.

1. Cultural differences – between the UK in general, and UK general practice in particular, and your home country. There is widespread acceptance that the CSA is not, nor should it be, a culturally neutral exam.
2. Expectation – of the role of patients and of doctors, both within the confines of the consultation and wider society.
3. Language – consulting outside of your native tongue is challenging for anyone, and if you then add in the colloquialisms that patients use for medical issues it is even more difficult.

We recognise that the journey for you as an OMG through GP training is likely to be more difficult than for a UK graduate, and so the primary aim of this book is to help you navigate that journey. We hope that through this book we will equip you to be a better UK general practitioner than you might otherwise be. An inevitable by-product of that will be improved success in postgraduate exams. Hopefully you will also experience the enhanced job satisfaction that comes from a sense of a job well done. You will also be better equipped to improve your own continuing professional development (CPD) and so provide better patient care, and satisfy the requirements of appraisal and revalidation.

In the UK the healthcare system is led by primary care and patients maintain a high level of trust in their GPs.[12,13] This means that as a GP you will need to be able to demonstrate a wide range of competencies, so it is worth looking at the professional competencies that form part of the MRCGP exam.[14] You might also find it helpful to review the professional competencies on which GP selection is based.[15] Some of these will be more difficult for those who qualified overseas, as the way in which they are demonstrated will be different from what might be expected in your country of origin. This is something that we will go into in much more detail in the remainder of this book, looking particularly at some of the linguistic and cultural aspects. However, we believe that recognising that this difference exists is one of the first steps in achieving success. After all, if you were training for the London Marathon you would take it rather more seriously than if you were aiming for the local 5 km charity fun run! If an expert personal trainer offered you some personalised support then you wouldn't turn it down – you would recognise that as being foolish. Yet, unfortunately, many overseas medical graduates still think that they can do it alone and ignore the expert help that is on offer to them. Others choose to put their faith in individuals who, while they are well motivated and keen to help, may not have the requisite expertise to provide sound advice. This book aims to be one way of providing such help and advice, but each GP school* is likely to have its own initiatives on offer that will complement it. This book is going to be peppered with ideas, or 'action points', for you to take forward and here is the first one.

ACTION POINT 1

- Find out what my local GP school offers as extra support for overseas medical graduates.
- If my GP school does not offer any proactive help, but rather waits until individuals fail, then campaign for this to change.

Accepting the help that is on offer to you is one of the first steps toward becoming an effective independent practitioner. However, sometimes GP schools, and individual trainers, can be nervous that offering such help can be perceived as being politically insensitive. You can help to avoid this by opening up the conversation and inviting them to share their ideas with you; perhaps you could even show them this book. After all, GP trainers are all successful UK general practitioners so, even if they trained before the advent of the current form of the MRCGP exam, they are well placed to give you guidance and support.

---

* With the advent of Health Education England, the terms relating to the organisations that provide GP training have changed and they are now officially called local education and training boards (abbreviated as LETBs). However, the terms 'deanery' and 'GP school' continue to remain in widespread use and are well recognised. Hence we have chosen to continue to use these terms throughout the book. GP school refers to the local provision of GP training, whereas deanery refers to the local provision of all specialty training, of which GP training is a part.

Sometimes trainers may say that they feel ill-equipped to help you. If this is the case then your GP school may well offer them some specific guidance, but it is also worth reminding them that they certainly do have a lot to offer you, as they have already achieved what you want to achieve – namely, becoming a UK general practitioner. Some OMGs find that working with a trainer who has come from overseas and managed to achieve success in the UK is the most beneficial. Others find that trainers who are originally from the UK have a better understanding of some of the more intriguing aspects of British language and culture. Both approaches have their pros and cons. The most important thing is finding someone with whom you can develop a good relationship.

We recognise, however, that accepting help is not always easy. There may also be cultural factors that make it even more difficult for some of you. We also realise that many of you may have been high-fliers in your home country and success has always come easily to you, so the possibility of failure seems an unlikely prospect. Focusing on this end point of becoming a fully qualified GP rather than the hurdles that you have to jump between now and then, such as the small matter of the MRCGP exam, may really help, for in that way you can see this as simply preparing sensibly for a change in your career progression. I (MF) prepare in a similar way when considering working overseas as part of my sabbaticals. I seek to find out as much as I can about the prevailing medical and general culture in the countries in which I plan to work. My colleagues have always seen this as sensible preparation, and it has not diminished my professional standing in any regard. For example, I have worked in Madagascar with rural tribal communities where they have a tradition of digging up their ancestors every 7 years and having a big party, where they all celebrate by having sex with one another to get rid of any evil spirits. This inevitably results in a large number of sexually transmitted infections, particularly gonorrhoea and chlamydia, with subsequent issues with pelvic inflammatory disease and infertility. Without knowing of this particular custom this would have been mystifying to me but, knowing that, it makes perfect sense. Within the UK we may not have such extreme examples but there are certainly idiosyncrasies that may not immediately be familiar to someone who has not grown up steeped in British culture.

Our hope is that this book will serve as a useful guide, with a menu of options for you to explore. Some will make sense, others less so. We would just encourage you to give them all a chance, as you never know where they might lead.

REFERENCES

1. Esmail A, Roberts C. *Independent Review of the Membership of the Royal College of General Practitioners (MRCGP) Examination.* Manchester: University of Manchester; 2013. Available at: www.gmc-uk.org/MRCGP_Final_Report__18th_September_2013. pdf_53516840.pdf (accessed 30 September 2013).

2. Patterson F, La-Band A, Koczwara A, *et al. GP National Selection Process: equalities impact.* Derbyshire: Work Psychology Group; 2012. Available at: www.gprecruitment. org.uk/reports/Equalities_Impact_Report.pdf (accessed 30 August 2013).

3. Esmail A, Roberts C. Academic performance of ethnic minority candidates and discrimination in the MRCGP examinations between 2010 and 2012: analysis of data. *BMJ.* 2013; **347**: f5662.

4. Dowling PT. Discrimination in the UK's postgraduate examination in primary care. *BMJ.* 2013; **347**: f5765.

5. Hawthorne K, Freeman A, Rughani A, *et al.* The Royal College of General Practitioners replies to the BMJ. *BMJ.* 2013; **347**: f5900.

6. Wakeford R. International medical graduates' relative under-performance in the MRCGP AKT and CSA examinations. *Educ Prim Care.* 2012; **23**(3): 148–52.

7. GMC faces high court action over pass rate discrepancy. Available at: http://bma. org.uk/news-views-analysis/news/2013/october/gmc-faces-high-court-action-over-exam-pass-rate-disparity (accessed 21 November 2013).

8. Denney ML, Freeman A, Wakeford R. MRCGP CSA: are the examiners biased, favouring their own by sex, ethnicity, and degree source? *Br J Gen Pract.* 2013; **63**(616): e718–25.

9. Tyrer SP, Leung W-C, Smalls J, *et al.* The relationship between medical school of training, age, gender and success in the MRCPsych examinations. *Psychiatr Bull.* 2002; **26**: 257–63.

10. Dewhurst NG, McManus C, Mollon J, *et al.* Performance in the MRCP(UK) Examination 2003–4: analysis of pass rates of UK graduates in relation to self-declared ethnicity and gender. *BMC Med.* 2007; **5**: 8.

11. Health and Social Care Information Centre – Workforce Directorate. *General and Personal Medical Services England 2002–2012.* 21-3-0013. Leeds: Health and Social Care Information Centre; 2013.

12. Kearley KE, Freeman GK, Heath A. An exploration of the value of the personal doctor-patient relationship in general practice. *Br J Gen Pract.* 2001; **51**(470): 712–18. Available at: www.ncbi.nlm.nih.gov/pmc/articles/PMC1314098/pdf/11593831.pdf (accessed 3 October 2013).

13. Tarrant C, Windridge K, Boulton M, *et al.* Research: qualitative study of the meaning of personal care in general practice. *BMJ.* 2003; **326**(7402): 1310–17. Available at: www.bmj.com/content/326/7402/1310.full (accessed 3 October 2013).

14. Royal College of General Practitioners (RCGP). WPBA competence framework. London: RCGP. Available at: www.rcgp.org.uk/gp-training-and-exams/mrcgp-workplace-based-assessment-wpba/wpba-competence-framework.aspx (accessed 3 October 2013).

15. National Health Service (NHS). *2014 Person Specification: general practice (ST1).* Available at: http://gprecruitment.hee.nhs.uk/downloads/2014-PS-GP-ST1-1.01.pdf (accessed 11 November 2013).

CHAPTER 1

Looking after yourself

Looking after yourself may not initially seem to be one of your main priorities when thinking about your GP training. However, before you rush to turn
to Chapter 5: Succeeding at Assessment, please stop for a minute and take the
time to read on. We firmly believe that actually taking care of yourself is one of
the cornerstones of achieving success. Ensuring that you look after your own
needs can make a real difference to your mindset, which in turn can enable you
to be much more open to the possibility of change. After all, becoming a GP
is not an easy process, but then neither is being a GP. Taking time to develop
good habits during your training will help to prevent later problems such as
professional isolation and burnout. Also, some of the strategies may even help
you to succeed at your GP training itself.

> It's not that simple or easy! It needed a lot of hard work, dedication, time management, team
> work, business skills and most importantly communication skills.
>
> Akansha

MONEY ISSUES

Although you have a reasonable salary as a GP specialty registrar (GPStR), the
costs associated with GP training are substantial. A number of these costs will
only come toward the end of your training, but they are entirely predictable so
it makes sense to budget for them throughout your 3-year training programme
so that you do not add running into debt to your potential stresses.

TABLE 1.1 Costs of becoming a general practitioner (at October 2013)

Item	Cost	Total	Link
Initial Associate in Training (AiT) subscription	£163	£1270	www.rcgp.org.uk/new_professionals/associates_in_training/fees.aspx
Annual AiT subscription	£369 × three for a 3-year programme		
Applied Knowledge Test (AKT) (with AiT discount)	£465	£465	
Clinical Skills Assessment (CSA) (with AiT discount)	£1563	£1563	
General Medical Council (GMC) registration	£390 per year	£1170	www.gmc-uk.org/doctors/fees.asp
Certificate of Completion of Training (CCT)	£390	£390	www.rcgp.org.uk/gp-training-and-exams/gp-certification-overview.aspx
	TOTAL	£4858	
	With two CSA attempts	£6421	

So that means you need to budget for a minimum of £125 per month, or £175 per month if you factor in the possibility of needing to resit your CSA exam. That is before you take into account any courses or study aids that you might also like to consider (although these may be reimbursable through your study allowance) and any travel costs associated with the exams. Factoring in potential extra costs, such as a second attempt at your CSA, makes sense, as it means that if you are unfortunate enough to need it then you won't have to also worry about the cost, whereas if you pass first time then you can celebrate by going on holiday!

It is also important to establish that you are on the right pay grade. This is particularly the case for overseas medical graduates, who often switch to general practice from other careers within the National Health Service (NHS), rather than entering GP training directly from the Foundation programme.

If you enter GP training from Foundation then you will be on pay grade StR00 (the minimum pay scale) at specialty training year 1 (St1), progressing up one point for each year so as to be StR01 at St2 and StR02 at St3. However, if you have undertaken 2 years, for example, of core surgical training before switching to GP then you will enter St1 at pay grade StR 02.

ACTION POINT 1

Check your payslip to see which pay grade you are on – is this accurate? What is your incremental date? (This is usually August but it may be different if you started in the NHS at some other time.)

It also makes sense to check that you are getting appropriately reimbursed for any expenses that you incur. If you are in a general practice setting then you can be reimbursed for travel expenses, including travel to and from work (for a maximum of 20 miles each way) provided that you use your car for business during the working day, such as undertaking a home visit. The forms for this should be available from your local GP training scheme or practice manager.

Similarly, if you have moved geographical area in order to undertake your GP training you may be eligible for help with removal expenses. The arrangements for claiming these vary between deaneries, so it is best to approach them directly to find out how the rules are applied in your local area.

Sometimes people undertake locums in order to supplement their income. For example, doing accident and emergency (A&E) locums at the weekend. If you are employed as a full-time GP trainee, then this is effectively moonlighting and requires the permission of your educational supervisor (ES), and often also your programme director (PD). Getting such agreement is not guaranteed, particularly if you are struggling with your GP training. If you are working on a less than full-time basis then it is usually not permitted to take on additional work.

It also has implications for the European Working Time Directive (abbreviated as EWTD),[1] which you can opt out of; however, it also affects clinical governance issues such as how safe and effective a practitioner you can be if you have been working for an excessively long period. Complaints are now unfortunately a common feature of general practice. It will be much harder to argue against such an event if it is discovered that you have been working excessive hours, even if you are personally confident that your clinical judgement was not affected by tiredness.

If you do undertake any additional work, even on a voluntary basis, you will need to declare this on Form R each year as part of your annual review of competence of progression (abbreviated as ARCP), as this now forms part of the mandatory requirements for revalidation. You will also be expected to get confirmation from whoever is supervising you in this additional role that you have not been involved in any serious untoward incidents or have any unresolved complaints.

If you are really struggling with financial issues then it is worth considering exploring what extra help you can get. The Royal Medical Benevolent Fund has access to various grants and a really useful website (www.support4doctors.org. uk). This covers a lot of different areas and signposts to other organisations that may be able to help.

It was bad enough failing my exam without having to humiliate myself by asking the bank manager for another loan.

Daniel

HOLIDAYS

Taking your annual leave entitlement is an important part of looking after yourself. So again, it is important to understand how many days' annual leave you are entitled to and plan early when you intend to take it.

ACTION POINT 2

Plan your annual leave at the beginning of each post – have you booked the time off work? Have you co-ordinated with your family?

In hospital posts it is sometimes challenging to be able to be completely flexible about when you take your leave. Indeed, many rotas include fixed holiday leave (although this is not recommended by the British Medical Association (BMA)) but actually being able to take your leave should not be an issue. If you find that it is, then you need to make early contact with your GP training PD to discuss the situation.

In general practice you will be supernumerary, so taking your annual leave should be much less of an issue. However, surgeries are often booked up to 6 weeks ahead, so you will be much more popular if you advise the practice manager of your intentions well in advance. If you already have full surgeries booked it would not be unreasonable of the practice to refuse your request, unless there are exceptional circumstances to explain the late notice.

SOMETHING TO THINK ABOUT

Are you better off taking regular blocks of 1 week of annual leave or do you ideally need 2 or more weeks to be able to properly switch off?

How much leave you are entitled to depends on which point of the pay scale you are on – *see* the section 'Money Issues' at the beginning of this chapter.
- Pay points StR00 to StR02 on the pay scale are entitled to 25 days' leave (i.e. most GP trainees who are moving from the Foundation programme).
- Pay point StR03 or higher on the pay scale is entitled to 30 days' leave (if you have some prior experience of specialty training and so enter GP training at a higher pay point).

You are also entitled to the eight annual bank holidays and, while in hospital posts, you will be entitled to two additional statutory NHS days' leave too. What this means is, regardless of your training grade, your holiday entitlement will go down by 2 days a year when you are in a general practice placement.

ACTION POINT 3

Check your contract of employment – have you been allocated the correct amount of annual leave?

FAITH AND WORK

Having a vibrant faith can be very sustaining in your everyday life. Indeed, lots of studies show that having religious convictions are good for you.[2-4] However, it can also lead to some potential conflicts in your professional life.[5] You can decrease the potential stress associated with this by thinking about some of these areas in advance to reduce their impact. This in no way compromises your ability to maintain your religious convictions, but it does enable you to think about how this relates to your professionalism. Communication is of key importance, as you cannot expect your trainer or PD to understand the potential significance of aspects of your faith. Most of them are willing to learn and issues usually only arise when there has been a lack of communication between all the interested parties.

For example, do you want to be able to attend communal prayers during Friday lunchtimes? If so, perhaps it is worth considering whether the practice that has its main clinical meeting on a Friday lunchtime is the right fit for you. Do you object to arranging terminations of pregnancy? Are you uncomfortable prescribing post-coital contraception? Or what about providing contraception to unmarried couples? If this is the case, then is a practice with a large element of student health well suited to you? If you do conscientiously object to certain clinical scenarios then it is worth telling your trainer and the receptionists at your GP practice, as then they can avoid booking patients in with you if they know in advance that is what the patient wants.

Clearly sometimes patients will present with requests that you are uncomfortable with, as the receptionists are not always aware of the reason for requesting a consultation. It is worth thinking about how you might approach such consultations so that they are still effective, patient-centred consultations. Things to think about would include how to explain your position without sounding judgemental of the patient's predicament, and also how you would signpost them to other routes of access for the services they need. Discussing this with your trainer would also be good preparation for your CSA. It should also provide evidence for a good reflective learning log entry about ethical issues and fitness to practise.

An example of how you might approach such an issue is as follows:

Miss J: I think I'm pregnant …
Doctor: What makes you think that? [*a non-judgemental statement that does not make any assumptions about how the patient might feel*]

Miss J: Well, my period is a fortnight late and I did a home pregnancy test which was positive.

Doctor: That suggests you are probably right. How do you feel about being pregnant? [*establishing the patient's thoughts about her situation*]

Miss J: I can't be pregnant. It's not the right time. I want a termination.

Doctor: Let's talk about that. Have you spoken to anyone else about the pregnancy? What about your partner? [*non-judgemental, finding out more about what the patient has already done/thought about*]

Miss J: It's none of his business. I just want to get rid of it and pretend it never happened.

Doctor: Pretending it never happened will be difficult. Have you had a termination before? [*continuing to be non-judgemental and finding out more background*]

Miss J: Of course not, I'm not stupid!

Doctor: What do you understand about your options? [*exploring if the patient understands what is available*]

Miss J: I don't want options. I just want a termination. Are you going to refer me or not?

Doctor: I'm afraid that my personal views mean that I don't agree with terminations. [*clear statement of fact*]

Miss J: Who do you think you are, telling me what is right and wrong!

Doctor: That is not what I am saying. If you are sure that you want a termination then I can refer you to one of my colleagues or to the pregnancy advisory service. I just want to be sure that you realise it is not your only option. [*not responding to the patient's anger, assuring the patient of your on-going care and arranging an alternative way that they can access care*]

Miss J: It is the only option for me.

Doctor: That may well be how it feels right now but you have time to think about what else might be possible. Do you think there is anyone you could talk to about this? [*continuing to explore options with the patient*]

Miss J: No, it's my body. I'll do what I like.

Doctor: I really would encourage you to confide in someone. But if you feel you can't, what about talking to the pregnancy advisory service? [*providing good clinical care and continuing to engage with the patient*]

Miss J: Will they give me a termination?

Doctor: Yes, if that is what you still want, after talking it through. [*enabling the patient to access alternative sources of medical care whilst maintaining your conscientious objection*]

Miss J: Can you refer me to them then?

Doctor: Yes I'll do that. Do you want to talk about anything else? What about contraception for the future? Have you given that any thought?

Being a GP is an enormous privilege but it does mean that you regularly come into contact with people whose lifestyles may be at odds with your own. Other areas that you might be less comfortable with are those relating to alcoholism, drug misuse, gambling issues, gender realignment or same-sex relationships. Thinking about such issues in advance can be really helpful. Inevitably, of course, it will sometimes be the unpredictable nature of consultations that catches you off guard!

ACTION POINT 4

Read the GMC guidance *Personal Beliefs and Medical Practice*[5] and think about what impact this will have on your clinical practice.

COMMUTING

Sometimes OMGs seem to find that they are commuting a significant distance to work. This seems to be more of an issue than for some of their colleagues and may relate to the fact that placements are often arranged in relation to performance at selection, so OMGs may well not get their first preference of geographical area. A significant commute at either end of the day can substantially add to your stress levels, so it is worth thinking about ways that you can try to reduce its impact. It will also inevitably eat into the time that you have available for studying, as well as relaxing with your family and friends. Different strategies will work for different individuals depending upon their particular circumstances, but it is worth trying to think creatively about how to improve the situation.

For example, could you leave home earlier so as to be able to miss the rush hour traffic and use the time you arrive before your surgery starts to do some revision or to catch up with your e-portfolio? Is it worth considering staying over nearer your workplace for a couple of nights a week? You could balance out the costs of accommodation with the money you will save on petrol, or perhaps even find a friend to stay with. You could also then use those evenings to concentrate on your GP training, doing revision or participating in a study group, so that for the nights that you are at home you can be fully available to your family.

You could also think about how to utilise your commute as a learning opportunity. For example, try listening to podcasts of learning modules, or from high-profile speakers such as the Chair of the Royal College of General Practitioners (RCGP). Or if English is not your first language then what about listening to spoken word radio, such as *The Archers* on BBC Radio 4? This will give you some fascinating insights into English culture as well as helping to improve your understanding and pronunciation.

Finally, if it is all getting too much, then seek help from your local GP training scheme. Do you have grounds for applying for an inter-deanery transfer?

What about an intra-deanery transfer? If you live at the edge of your local training scheme's area do they actually know this? If not, then you can hardly complain when you are expected to travel across the area to a distant practice. Is there scope for reducing your working hours? There may be little flexibility within the hospital components of your rotations but within general practice it *may* be possible to work 4 long days, for example. If you do not ask then you will never know what you might be able to arrange.

> Being an IMG [international medical graduate] I never knew that I could go for part-time training, as I was struggling with my home life. There was no closeness with my programme directors in this regard and no formal ways to assess the trainee's level of stress. I was sent to a new trainer to try new strategies far away from my home. I was so desperate to pass my exam I agreed to any kind of hardship.
>
> Shahida

Arranging an intra-deanery transfer is at the discretion of your own deanery, and the criteria can vary. However, the essential premise is that there has to have been a material change in your circumstances since you started your GP training. Examples might include your partner relocating, a new baby or personal or family illness. Similar principles apply for inter-deanery transfers, but these are now centrally organised by the London Deanery. The exact requirements can be found online (www.londondeanery.ac.uk/var/idt). However, it is worth remembering that, even if you have good reasons for applying for a transfer that are found to fulfil the necessary criteria, whether you actually get to move deanery depends upon whether where you want to move to has any room for you! This varies between areas, as clearly some, such as London, are more popular than others. There are also strict timescales for applying, with two transfer windows each year, so if this is something that interests you then look at the available information early.

WORK–LIFE BALANCE

Obviously, regular holidays are a key part of your work–life balance, but this is also something that you need to review regularly. Being a doctor is not the only role that is important in your life: you will also be a son or daughter, friend and colleague. You may also be a husband or wife, or mum or dad. Taking time to sustain these relationships will play a key role in maintaining your work–life balance.

Hopefully these relationships will be ones that sustain you through your GP training and support you through any difficulties. Sometimes, however, you will be the one needing to support others in your life. Perhaps you have an elderly father whose health is deteriorating? Or perhaps you are preparing to get married? Or perhaps you are even facing the prospect of treatment for infertility? Or are you learning how to combine work with the arrival of a new baby? Often GP training coincides with times of significant life change. Again communication is crucial, as you cannot expect others to support you if you are relying on their psychic abilities to know that you need help. Sometimes different cultures place different emphases on the role of family in particular situations. Your PD or ES may not immediately realise this and so may be at risk of underestimating the degree of stress that a situation puts you under, unless you explain this to him or her.

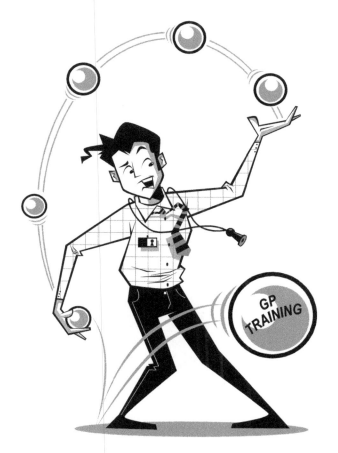

However, compartmentalisation can also help to some extent. Is there some way perhaps that you can identify certain times that you will be fully available to your family? Perhaps you will agree not to work on Sundays or just to do 2 hours on Saturday. Could you get up an hour or two earlier at the weekend and do a small burst of studying before concentrating on your family's needs? Obviously, there will still inevitably be the odd crisis that eats into this pattern but hopefully that will be the exception rather than the norm. Trying to be proactive rather than simply reacting to events as they occur is a good way of reducing your stress levels.

So is building in time for yourself, as an individual, rather than in one of your other roles. What do you enjoy? Is it going to the gym, or playing golf? Reading? Art? If you are going to feel guilty about this then you could even incorporate it into your learning activities. Joining a book club will improve your English conversation skills. Starting an evening pottery or woodwork class will improve your manual dexterity and also bring you into contact with a whole new subset of English society. The best GPs are well-rounded individuals with life outside the consulting room! You are more than a doctor, you are you, so find out what recharges your batteries and makes you tick!*

There are various tools available that can help to challenge you as to whether the balance in your life is right. One of those used commonly is the Wheel of Life,[6] which enables you to take a step back and look at your life from above, as if from a helicopter. How this works is that you look at each of the spokes and rank where your life is currently (not where you think it should be!) from 1 to 10. Then try joining all your spokes together. If this creates a wheel would it be a bumpy ride? What can you do to make it smoother? Are there any areas that need urgent attention in your life?

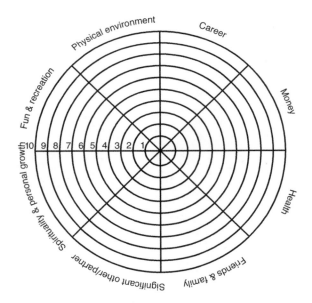

FIGURE 1.1 Wheel of Life

Doing such an exercise can sometimes be challenging, so you might like to think about whether there is someone you could discuss the results with. This could be a professional colleague, a family member or even a mentor. It can also help you to think about how the spokes are inter-related. For example, you might conclude that you are spending too much time on work but you are happy with the money that you currently earn. If locums in A&E are supplementing your income then, obviously, stopping these will improve your work balance but it will potentially have a negative impact on your money spoke. So you will need to try to decide which of these is your priority! You might also identify that at the moment your family is suffering but recognise that this is probably a consequence of the fact that your CSA is approaching. This might mean that you do not feel able to adjust things at the moment but you could make plans for the future, such as arranging a family holiday soon after the exam. Recognising such issues, even if you are unable to immediately change them, can have a really positive effect on your stress levels.

ACTION POINT 5

- Formally take some time (probably at least half an hour) to look at your work–life balance, using a tool such as the Wheel of Life if you find that helpful. Is it in balance? Are there any areas that need reviewing urgently?
- Share your thoughts with your family – do they agree? Do they have any suggestions to help change the situation?

SICK LEAVE

Some of you will inevitably find that you become unwell during your training. This can range from obvious physical ailments, such as breaking your leg on a skiing holiday, to mental health issues that can lead to protracted time off work. Doctors, as a group, are more susceptible to mental health issues than the general population[7-10] and these can become even more prevalent for someone facing difficulties in their professional life, often for the first time. Developing mental health issues is nothing to be ashamed of and it is much better to face up to this reality than taking an ostrich approach* of putting your head in the sand and hoping it will go away.

> I am very depressed now and have lost all my hope. I am on sick leave and waiting to recover and go back to work.
>
> Haroun

Ensuring that you have good support networks, including being appropriately registered with a GP local to where you live, is essential in helping you in the

---

Phrase notes
* 'ostrich approach' – refusing to accept reality or recognise the truth

face of such difficulties. So is recognising when your work is at risk of suffering, as a consequence of your health issues. As far as your GP training is concerned, either you are fit to be at work and expected to continue with the requirements of workplace-based assessment (WPBA) or you are not fit for work. There is no halfway house whereby you can continue to fulfil your clinical duties but not continue your ongoing training. However, there are alternatives that you can access with the help of occupational health and your PD team. This might include a phased return to work following an episode of illness or perhaps being temporarily excused from working nights. As with everything else, what matters is early communication about your difficulties rather than trying to struggle on regardless.

Taking time off sick will affect your training but far less than facing a complaint or serious untoward incident that has far-reaching consequences for you and your patients. Any unscheduled leave that you take (which could include sick leave and compassionate leave, for example) that is more than 14 days of rostered work in any 12-month period will need to be made up. However, you only need to make up the time that you lose, so if you end up having 6 weeks off work your training will be extended by a month. The only exception to this might be if you are undertaking a post of short duration. Although general practice training is now competency rather than time based, any posts that are shorter than 3 months' duration are likely to be more scrutinised. So there will need to be evidence of their educational value in your e-portfolio in order for them to count toward your training. Liaising early with your GP training scheme should make this a relatively straightforward process. So make sure that they are aware of the situation and that you provide copies of any sick notes to the deanery so that your e-portfolio accurately reflects your current situation. After all, the last thing you need when depressed is someone chasing you for not keeping up to date with your learning log!

Recognising your stress early can, however, avoid the need for lengthy periods of sick leave (for some individuals) and, as always, prevention is far better than cure. Try talking to your family and friends and giving them permission to tell you if they think that you are struggling. Try to notice for yourself how you are feeling – do you always struggle to sleep on Sunday night for fear of work on Monday mornings? Are you losing the ability to enjoy yourself? Are you starting to have difficulty with seeing patients as people rather than as objects? Then, having recognised these traits, take action. Some studies[9] have shown that it is the 'perception of stress' rather than stress itself that makes individuals at risk of burnout, so just because your colleagues sailed through[*] their busy paediatric job does not mean that you will do the same.

Some people have difficulty with this concept; if this is you, then you might

---

Phrase notes
* 'sailed through' – to achieve something with little apparent effort

like to explore some of the external support organisations available to you. The Doctors' Support Network is a self-help group of doctors dealing with mental health issues and offers an online discussion forum as well as a telephone helpline.[11] Similarly, the BMA offers a telephone-based counselling service.[12] There may also be local support services that you can access via your deanery, so do talk to your programme director team.

> I never thought I would be the one to struggle. After all I had sailed through everything, I was one of the youngest to pass PACES [part 2 of the exams for Membership of the Royal College of Physicians]. So it all came as a bit of a shock. I ended up off work, which might not have been needed if I had listened to my family.
>
> Shaneil

Hopefully this chapter has given you some practical advice about how to look after yourself and minimise the likelihood of problems arising during your GP training. The key message is *early communication*, before things get out of hand. Most deaneries have some sort of professional support organisation that can offer you a variety of help, such as mentoring support, linguistic input or even psychotherapy, depending on your particular needs. Your GP training team will know how to access this, so it is worth talking to them early.

> I didn't know that the Career Development Unit existed until I talked to my programme director. Thinking back I should have picked up on the warning signs earlier. Who knows what difference that would have made!
>
> Eleanor

Finally, it is worth trying to keep a positive outlook on life. Try to keep any setbacks in perspective. Find out what nurtures you and then do it! Give yourself permission to be selfish on occasion. Turn your daydreams into reality …

> All men dream: but not equally. Those who dream by night in the dusty recesses of their minds wake in the day to find that it was vanity: but the dreamers of the day are dangerous men, for they may act their dreams with open eyes, to make it possible.
>
> TE Lawrence (Lawrence of Arabia), *Seven Pillars of Wisdom*

REFERENCES

1. *European Working Time Directive*. Leeds: NHS Employers; 2011. Available at: www.nhsemployers.org/PlanningYourWorkforce/MedicalWorkforce/EWTD/Pages/EWTD.aspx (accessed 23 October 2013).
2. Matthews DA, Larson DB, Barry CP. *The Faith Factor: an annotated bibliography of clinical research on spiritual subjects*. Rockville, MD: John Templeton Foundation, National Institute for Healthcare Research; 1994.
3. Levin JS. Religion and health: is there an association, is it valid, and is it causal? *Soc Sci Med*. 1994; **38**(11): 1475–82.
4. Matthews DA, McCullough ME, Larson DB, *et al*. Religious commitment and health status: a review of the research and implications for family medicine. *Arch Fam Med*. 1998; **7**(2): 118–24.
5. General Medical Council (GMC). *Personal Beliefs and Medical Practice (2013)*. London: GMC; 2013. Available at: www.gmc-uk.org/guidance/ethical_guidance/21171.asp (accessed 2 May 2013).
6. Kersley SE. *Prescription for Change: for doctors who want a life*. Oxford: Radcliffe Publishing; 2006.
7. Caplan RP. Stress, anxiety, and depression in hospital consultants, general practitioners, and senior health service managers. *BMJ*. 1994; **309**(6964): 1261–3.
8. Sotile WM, Sotile MO. *The Resilient Physician*. Chicago, IL: American Medical Association; 2002.
9. Jones P, editor. *Doctors as Patients*. Oxford: Radcliffe Publishing; 2005.
10. McCranie EW, Brandsma JM. Personality antecedents of burnout among middle-aged physicians. *Behav Med*. 1988; **14**(1): 30–6.
11. www.dsn.org.uk
12. British Medical Association (BMA) Counselling Service. *Doctors' Well-Being*. London: BMA. Available at: http://bma.org.uk/practical-support-at-work/doctors-well-being/about-doctors-for-doctors (accessed 23 October 2013).

CHAPTER 2

Learning how to learn

Learning how to learn is the next part of the journey to becoming a GP that we want to concentrate on. This is not only about passing all the assessments along the way (although that is obviously important) but also about preparing yourself for your CPD once you are qualified. With the advent of revalidation, being able to demonstrate how you keep up to date is becoming increasingly important, so it makes sense to get into good habits when you are training.

The first step toward effective learning is about ensuring that you are in the right frame of mind to be able to take on board new ideas and knowledge.

Maslow,[1] a humanist psychologist, talks about having a hierarchy of needs.

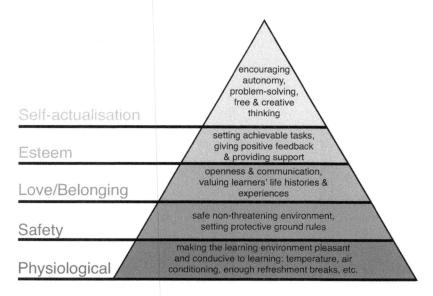

FIGURE 2.1 Maslow's hierarchy of needs

Like all models this one is not perfect, and it is certainly open to criticism as being based on a very individual view of society. However, we would argue that we can certainly recognise truth in the idea that if you have not sorted out your basic needs then you will not be in a good position to think about other issues – about becoming who you were born to be.* We have tried to cover most of these elements in the previous chapter, which is why we felt that was an important place to start. If you are struggling at an emotional level then it will be hard to take on any constructive feedback as to how you might change without it damaging your self-esteem. You may also find that your trainer becomes more reluctant to even give you such feedback for fear of upsetting you, which will not be helpful in the longer term in helping you develop.

It is also worth considering the environment in which you undertake your learning. Do you study best at home or at work? Why is that? What are the main distractions to your learning? How could you address these? Given that we find that patients are a rich source of learning material for most people, you may like to consider how you could improve your consulting room, as this is where you will spend a large proportion of your time. Getting some plants, some pictures or even some photos of your family may really help with your motivation. It may also have the added benefit of helping patients to feel more at ease, which will result in enhanced communication.

Finally, it is worth being honest with your trainer or clinical supervisor (CS) about where you are on this hierarchy. You cannot expect them to be sympathetic to your situation if they do not know about it. If you are struggling financially, or worried about a family member far away, or losing sleep because your child has colic then this is likely to impact on your educational performance. If your trainer understands this then, although they cannot change the goalposts that need to be achieved, they may be able to work with you to come up with some helpful strategies. At the very least it will enable them to show more empathy toward you, rather than making assumptions that you are lazy and not motivated to learn. When it works well, the trainer–registrar relationship is one of the most powerful influences on your performance, and often results in lifelong friendships. So it is worth taking time to invest in this, and enabling your trainer to see you as an individual. All too often it is only when people are failing that some of the reasons behind this come to light, by which time it is often too late to do anything about it. This is so easily avoided if you can manage to have a good relationship with your ES and GP training team.

BECOMING AN ADULT LEARNER

All of my educational colleagues will be able to tell you that the word 'deliver' is one of my (MF) least favourite words in the English language. That is with reference to GP training and education; when I am ordering a pizza then I

Phrase notes
* 'born to be' – to strongly show a particular quality or behaviour

hope for prompt, accurate delivery as much as the next person! However, in the context of education the word delivery implies that you, the learner, are a passive receiver of information. This is 'child learning', where the agenda is the teacher's, and the teacher takes the responsibility for making decisions about what, how and when things will be learnt. This is the approach that is often taken in a school setting, at least some of the time, and also in undergraduate study. This is true of some English medical schools but seems to be particularly true of the experience of some OMGs in their home countries. Unfortunately this approach can only get you so far, and so postgraduate study, such as GP training, often focuses on more adult forms of learning. In educational speak, this means that there is a shift from 'pedagogy' (child learning) toward 'andragogy' (adult learning). Although even then some elements of pedagogy remain – for example, in very structured educational sessions such as an advanced life support (ALS) course.

Neither approach is 'right' or 'wrong' but the reality is that when the curriculum you need to cover is as huge as that involved in GP training, there needs to be a significant proportion of learner-led, or adult, learning, or you will have no hope of covering all of the material that you need to. The MRCGP exam uses the principles of adult education, with its focus on reflection and learning from experience, which is also advocated by the GMC.[2] It is also the approach that you will need to take once you have completed your training in order to demonstrate your commitment to your ongoing professional development and fulfil the requirements of revalidation. Additionally, in lots of people's opinions, it is a more interesting way of fulfilling your learning needs. It means that you can target your learning toward what you need, or want, to find out more about.

> Here my learning technique has changed. It is more case-based learning guidelines and help in management. Peer discussion is also very helpful.
>
> Gloria

> My learning in GP training is self-directed. I need to read about conditions soon after seeing them or at least write the condition's name and a few details that I remember down. Not all the required information is in one textbook.
>
> Katya

FINDING OUT HOW YOU PREFER TO LEARN

We are all different and so we all tend to prefer to learn and take on board new information in different ways. One of our PD colleagues tends to download podcasts and listen to them while doing the washing up, whereas others would much rather read a summary of the latest National Institute for Health and

Care Excellence (NICE) guidance or attend a study group where they can discuss clinical cases that the guidance is relevant to. Finding out how you prefer to learn can be really helpful in motivating you to learn, while recognising that sometimes circumstances, or the type of information that you need to acquire, may mean that you need to use a less preferred method some of the time. For example, it may well be that our colleague would also value attending a study group but is precluded from doing so by the time constraints of balancing a busy clinical workload with a family of three young children.

There are several different models of looking at how you learn best, but two of the most useful are the VARK model[3] and the Honey and Mumford Learning Styles,[4] which is derived from Kolb's learning cycle,[5] which we will come to later.

VARK MODEL[3,6]

The VARK acronym stands for visual, aural, read/write and kinaesthetic sensory modes of learning information. It was derived from the work of an American psychologist, Howard Gardner, who first described seven intelligences.[6] This suggests that each of us has a preferred way of learning and taking on board new information. That does not mean of course that we do not use other styles, either by choice or by necessity, and most people are using a mixture of learning styles all the time. However, spending some time thinking about your learning style may help you if you are having difficulty managing the demands of getting to grips with your GP training. It may also help to reassure you if you are finding the e-portfolio a challenge – that does not necessarily mean that you are failing or stupid, it may simply reflect the fact that verbal learning does not come as easily to you. This is also often the case when you are trying to complete a verbal learning task in your non-native tongue.

ACTION POINT 1

Consider using an online questionnaire to help you work out what your preferred learning style is (check out www.learning-styles-online.com).

Having established what your preferred learning style is, think about how you can make use of this information in helping you to consolidate your learning. It may also help to discuss this with your colleagues and find out who else in your cohort thinks in a similar way, as you may then be able to share learning resources.

Learning style	Preferences	Typical phrases
Visual (spatial)	Prefer using pictures, images and spatial understanding	Let's look at this differently … Let's see how this works for you … Let me draw you a diagram …
Aural (auditory–musical)	Prefer using sound or music	That sounds about right … That rings a bell … Tune in to what I'm saying …
Verbal (linguistic)	Prefer using words in speech and writing	Tell me word for word … Let me spell it out for you … Let's talk later …
Physical (kinaesthetic)	Prefer using your body, hands and sense of touch	My gut is telling me … I follow your drift … Get in touch with …
Logical (mathematic)	Prefer using logic and reasoning systems	There's no pattern to this … Let's make a list … Follow the rules …
Social (interpersonal)	Prefer to learn in groups or with other people	Help me to understand this … Let's pull together on this … Let's explore our options …
Solitary (intrapersonal)	Prefer to work alone and self-study	I'd like some time to think it over … Let me get back to you on that …

Visual learners

- Try using mind maps as a way of recording information. You can either hand draw these or investigate the numerous IT-based solutions that exist.
- Have multiple-coloured pens to highlight important aspects of information, such as when trying to revise NICE guidance.
- Use revision guides that include pictures and diagrams, not just bullet points of information.
- Familiarise yourself with multimedia approaches to learning, such as BMJ Learning, which may include video podcasts.
- Use diagrams when trying to explain things to patients – practise drawing simple schematics of things you might need to explain, such as the chambers of the heart, or the reproductive system – this may be particularly helpful if you regularly find that you struggle with this aspect of the consultation.

Aural learners

- Use rhythm and rhyme to help you create mnemonics of things that you need to remember. (We are sure you can probably still remember some of

these from medical school, although they may well be too rude to repeat in public!)
- Download podcasts to listen to.
- Record yourself reading out important topics and then listen to these in the car when travelling to and from work.
- Familiarise yourself with some sounds or music that soothe you and practise being able to recall this so that you can use it as an anchoring technique when under stress, such as when taking exams.

Verbal learners
- The e-portfolio was made for you, so use it regularly as a reflective tool.
- Use textbooks that are well written (like this one, hopefully!), not just bullet point summaries.
- Practise with colleagues through role playing.
- Consider recording yourself reading out familiar topics but try to vary your tone, making it more like a dramatic presentation.

Physical learners
- Try to use movement as much as possible in your learning.
- Consider using flashcards that you can then move around or draw out of a hat (the CSA case cards were made for you!).
- Don't just think about how you would undertake a physical examination, actually practise it with friends or colleagues.
- Use certain actions to tag thoughts and processes – for example, use the act of taking someone's blood pressure to prompt you into remembering the NICE recommendations as to which anti-hypertensive agent to use and when.
- Try using large pieces of paper to draw diagrams or mind maps, or list bullet points.

Logical learners
- Use textbooks that explain the rationale behind a particular management strategy – for example, rather than learning a rote list of which anti-hypertensive to use and when, think about the underlying physiology as to why a particular choice might be more appropriate.
- Try making associations between systems to think of the wider picture – for example, you could think about how you might consult with a patient with Down's syndrome, from the perspective of how you approach communicating with someone with a learning disability, and link this to the common medical complications that they might face, or the time management skills that you need for such complex interactions.
- Try not to overanalyse everything so much that you are paralysed by indecision – sometimes you just have to get on with it.

KOLB'S LEARNING CYCLE[5]

Kolb produced a description as to how adults learn. So for example if we think about the following consultation, with Jane, which serves as a springboard for learning:

An actual experience:

This consultation with Jane, a 43-year-old who has recently been diagnosed with secondaries from her breast cancer, is going really badly. I have no idea what to say to her.

Reflecting on what happened:

I found it difficult to talk to Jane because it was all so sad, knowing that she wouldn't see her young family grow up and have children of their own. I also realised that I was going to be running really, really late!

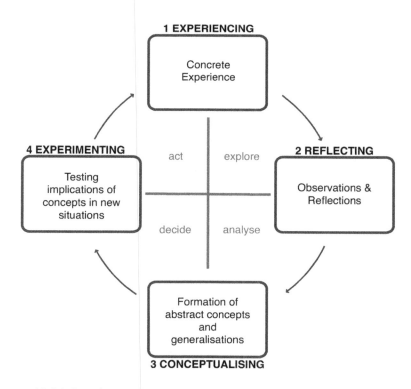

FIGURE 2.2 Kolb's learning cycle

Thinking about why this happened and how you might improve for next time:

I need to be able to separate myself from these sad situations, while still maintaining empathy, or I am going to burn out really quickly! I think I will always find it a challenge not to get too over-involved with patients and maybe this is something I need to talk about with my trainer.

I could ease the stress of running late by arranging to see patients who I know will take longer at the end of surgery, or allocating extra time for them.

Trying out your improvements:

I arranged to see Jane at the end of my surgery and we focused on the here and now and how she is feeling. I was less stressed, as there weren't any patients waiting, and we had a really inspiring conversation about her 'bucket list'* of things she wants to do before she dies. I felt less helpless, as I was also able to signpost her to support organisations for preparing her children for her death.

You can enter the learning cycle at any point. Sometimes it will be the practical experience of a consultation, as already described. Another time it might be reflection following a discussion with your colleagues about how to approach breaking bad news in the future. However, you are likely to have a preference for a particular aspect of the learning cycle, which is how Honey and Mumford[4] developed their learning styles.

Honey and Mumford Learning Styles
- Activists like to do, act or EXPERIENCE
- Reflectors like to explore, review or REFLECT
- Theorists like to analyse, theorise or CONCEPTUALISE
- Pragmatists like to plan, decide or EXPERIMENT.

FIGURE 2.3 The four learning styles

Activists

Activists like to be involved in new experiences and are enthusiastic about new ideas. They like being in the here and now.† They are good at coming up with new ideas but may not be able to follow through with implementing them. If this is you, then you might well benefit from exposing yourself to new experiences such as attending commissioning meetings with a view to thinking about the organisational aspects of general practice, rather than trying to read about it. You will probably find the reflective nature of the e-portfolio is not a good fit with your preferred method of learning, as you tend not to reflect on experiences after they have happened. You may also find that by the time you come to write an entry you have already fulfilled the learning need that you

---

Phrase notes

* 'bucket list' – list of things that someone wants to do before he or she dies or 'kicks the bucket'

† 'in the here and now' – in the present moment

identified, such as reading the relevant NICE guidance. However, you could think creatively about how you could do some further 'trying out' as a way of addressing further learning needs that you have identified. Role-playing situations with colleagues could be really useful for you.

Reflectors

In some ways GP training was designed for you, particularly with the new emphasis on reflection in WPBA. Being able to think about situations that you encounter will be really helpful in enabling you to make sense of uncertainty. Being able to deal with uncertainty is one of the cornerstones of general practice; particularly as more and more of what was previously our core workload is diverted to other healthcare practitioners such as practice nurses. You will probably learn well on your own; however, within a group setting you may have really useful insights as to why something did or didn't work, provided that the group are able to wait for you to talk.

Theorists

Theorists like to think through things in a logical process and understand the principles behind them. They can be uncomfortable with uncertainty in some situations. However, they may enjoy thinking laterally about situations once they can work out the relevance of it to the matter in hand. If this is you, then you may find the more pragmatic approach of some of your colleagues frustrating as you seek to learn more deeply about a particular subject. You would prefer structured teaching sessions with clear objectives and you may find that e-learning suits you well. You may find that you struggle with covering the breadth of knowledge needed for general practice and so you will need to balance your desire for understanding the intricacies of a particular subject with covering the spread of the curriculum.

Pragmatists

GPs are generally good pragmatists. The overriding principle is 'does it work?' The majority of GPs are not keen on lengthy theoretical discussions and are very practical and down to earth. If this is you then you will be comfortable with learning that is directly applicable to your job. So you might like case discussions of how to approach anti-hypertensive medications for particular patient groups rather than a discussion about the underlying physiology. You like being able to try out new techniques, so videoing your consultations and seeing what interventions work, and which don't, would be a good learning opportunity for you. Once you are in practice you will tend to be good at implementing things that you can see have a tangible benefit for your patients or give you some financial reward.

ACTION POINT 2

Can you work out who the activists, pragmatists, reflectors and theorists are in your practice team? What makes you think that? Can you identify what their strengths and weaknesses are? What would you say about them on a multi-source feedback (MSF)?

THE DOWNSIDES OF LEARNING STYLES

Considering your learning style can be a useful exercise in helping you to make sense of what ways of learning are best suited to you. They can help you to think outside the box* to look at different strategies, such as using sound and movement. However, as already explained, they are only preferences and so you should not dismiss learning opportunities that do not seem to immediately fit with your identified style. Most people in fact have a mix of preferences, which seems to be related not only to personality but also to exposure to different styles. For example, if you had a really inspirational teacher who concentrated on an activist approach then this might lead you to think more about activist ways of learning than you might otherwise do. Also it is worth remembering that throughout your career you will be expected to learn in ways that might not come as naturally to you. For example, it is now generally accepted that the ability to be able to reflect is crucial for most professional groups in ensuring that they are able to recognise their limitations and address their learning needs. So reflection is one of the main building blocks of revalidation as well as of your GP training, so you need to get used to it.

Learning styles are, however, a useful way of increasing your self-awareness, which can only be a positive thing. Another useful way of improving your self-awareness is that of getting feedback.

THE VALUE OF FEEDBACK

Failing an exam, such as your AKT or CSA, is one way of getting feedback but it is a pretty harsh way! What would be better would be to seek feedback as you progress through your training, in a developmental (otherwise known as formative) way so that you can try to improve. If you seek feedback in this way then you will have a chance to try out new strategies to see if they help, and seek further feedback, so completing the Kolb learning cycle.

Two Americans, Joey Luft and Harry Ingham,[7] came up with an interesting pictorial representation of the purpose of feedback, known as the Johari window (*see* Figure 2.4).

Phrase notes
* 'to think outside the box' – to think freely and creatively, not bound by any rules or expectations

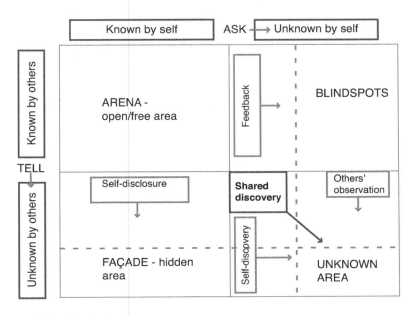

FIGURE 2.4 The Johari window

The purpose of getting feedback is to decrease your blind spots by enabling others to show you things about yourself that you are not currently aware of. However, before we go on to look at that in more detail, it is worth just thinking about the 'façade box' for a minute or two. It is generally accepted that what we are in fact aiming to do is to increase the size of the 'arena' box. If you look at Figure 2.4 you will see that reducing blind spots is one way of doing that (via feedback) but so is reducing the size of the façade. This involves you, as the learner, disclosing facts about yourself that your trainer may not be aware of. Helping them to understand you as an individual can really help in moving you forward. It may even help them to target their feedback more effectively. For OMGs this may include disclosing something about your cultural background, heritage and family situation.

> I worked in a small hospital (as an O&G [obstetrics and gynaecology] specialist) in northern Baghdad for 3 months. I could not stay there any longer. The hospital had no facilities available, very limited medications and no theatre after 2 p.m. so all patients in potential labour had to go to a nearby larger district hospital. All these were in addition to taking the risk of passing armed forces in the street on the way to work and getting killed by mistake. I decided it was time to leave my country for all sorts of reasons.
>
> Abdaal

Enabling your trainer to understand some of these background issues will really help them to get a sense of who you are and what motivates you, as well as what stresses you. Sometimes also talking about such issues can even help you to work out for yourself important issues that then decrease the size of your blind spot. For example, is Abdaal, quoted here, actually hankering after his original career choice of obstetrics that he felt forced to leave? If so, would he benefit from finding opportunities that help him to feel that such experiences were not wasted? Or is he worrying about family members and friends who may still live in Iraq?

ACTION POINT 3

Think about your life using the Johari window. How big is the façade box? Are there important areas or background issues that you have chosen not to share with your trainer? Why is that? Is it something you could change?

It is also worth remembering that feedback is a two-way process. So if you think your ES could do better in some regard, or, alternatively, if you found a particular approach worked really well for you, then it is worth telling him or her. After all, they too are keen to develop and they are also motivated by wanting you to do well.

How to give and receive effective feedback

Within your GP training there are several formal methods of achieving feedback about your performance from your colleagues and your patients as part of WPBA. This can be really useful in demonstrating how individuals who relate to you in different ways perceive you, if you compare the feedback that you get from different sources. Perhaps you can see different themes developing, depending upon whether it is your supervisor, your peer or a patient who is providing the feedback? However, it is always worth seeking continuing feedback throughout your training outside of these formal mechanisms.

There are several principles as to how to use feedback effectively, both as giver and receiver, and we will touch on these here.

- Remember that the purpose of feedback is to improve performance, so there is no point in being overly harsh or critical, as this has the potential to backfire and cause the person receiving the feedback to lose his or her motivation to change. Good feedback usually encompasses both positive and negative aspects, often with the development areas sandwiched in the middle. However, if someone really does need to improve significantly, don't concentrate so much on the positives that the negative aspects get lost completely or are easy to ignore! Once you know someone well it can really help to give them permission to concentrate on those areas that you need to develop further. This is what we have contracted to do in the learning set that we run specifically for OMGs, as it maximises the educational impact of a time-limited session. It can, however, come across as quite negative and demoralising, which is why you need to jointly agree to this approach if you think it would be helpful.
- Feedback is best done in a timely fashion. So if you are doing a joint surgery, for example, it would be good to be able to debrief between patients, or at the latest at the end of the surgery, rather than waiting until your tutorial time a week later. This means that the feedback will not be surprising, as you will be expecting it. It will also mean that you will be able to remember the specific examples that are given of areas where there is potential for change.
- Feedback is best given regularly. Obviously, if you only get feedback sporadically then it is much harder for it to be timely. However, giving it regularly also has the added benefit that you can start to think about what effect any small changes that you have made has had on the situation, or your performance. In this way you can constantly refine your development, testing out new ideas and making adjustments to your plans. Sometimes making a small change in one area can lead to unexpected negative consequences in another area and having regular feedback can help you to identify this at an early stage before your new habits become engrained and so more difficult to change.

- Specific feedback is much more helpful than generalisations. This will really help you to identify areas for change. It also usually forces the person giving the feedback to concentrate on what they know of you first-hand rather than relying on other people's ideas and viewpoints. Ideally it should include both specific observations and also specific suggestions as to what can be improved. It concentrates on *how* you achieved something as well as what you managed to achieve.
- Being able to attribute feedback to a particular situation can be really illuminating in trying to work out why something did (or didn't) work. That is why there is considerable debate among educationalists as to whether it is preferable to have feedback that is anonymous (as in your MSF as part of WPBA) or feedback that is attributable to a specific individual. Anonymising feedback can free people up to make constructive criticisms that they would not feel able to give face-to-face, particularly in situations of power imbalance such as employee–employer relationships. However, it can mean that the individual receiving the feedback struggles to make sense of it. For example, when I (MF) got some feedback from my practice that 'I could be grumpy', it made much more sense when it became clear that the feedback came from the particular receptionist who is on the front desk when I am duty doctor, as this is a situation that I can find quite stressful.
- Feedback needs to be handled sensitively, so think about the setting before launching in. None of us like to be criticised in public so try to find an appropriate place for giving and receiving feedback. This also means not trying to catch your supervisor in the corridor, as that may influence the quality of the feedback you get. By setting regular times to give and receive feedback you can decrease the need, and temptation, to catch people on the hop.*

There are some models of giving feedback that are regularly used within GP training and which can sometimes help, particularly in avoiding the tendency in all of us to leap to judging one another. If you are interested in finding out more about these then talk to your trainer or PD, but we will touch on two of the common ones here.

Phrase notes

* 'catch people on the hop' – to ask someone for something when they are not ready for it and so may not be able to deal with it well

PENDLETON'S PRINCIPLES

Pendleton *et al.*[8] concentrate on *providing challenge in a sea of support*. They concentrate on why some things have gone well whereas others have been less successful. One important aspect of this approach is that it is for use in conjunction with explicit standards. So it might work well, for example, when you are preparing for your CSA if your trainer gives you feedback based on the level you will need to reach in each of the domains in order to pass the exam.

Pendleton's approach has the following elements, which do not necessarily need to be performed in this order.

- **Contracting**: agree a time frame for the discussion, both the learner's and the teacher's agendas, roles and responsibilities.
- **Clarify** any matters of fact.
- **What the 'performer' did well**: get the person receiving the feedback to describe what he or she did well. This should concentrate on the performer's actions and what he or she did that resulted in a good outcome, rather than simply describing the outcome.
- **What the mentor thought the 'performer' did well**: ideally, the mentor will not simply agree with the performer but may be able to help tease out what it was that made a particular action effective, as well as identify other action points that the performer hasn't noticed for him- or herself.
- **What the 'performer' recommends for change**: this is the beginning of identifying opportunities for improvement and developing an action plan.
- **What the mentor recommends for change**: this again may include agreeing with, and refining, the performer's ideas, as well as adding new suggestions.

SET-GO APPROACH[9]

This approach also concentrates on objective statements of what is seen or heard, rather than making judgements, which are often not well received.

- *What did you See?* Explain what you (the trainee) saw or experienced.
- *What Else?* The trainer probes a little further to find out what else happened. What happened next? Did anyone else see what happened? What did he or she (your trainer) see?
- *What do you Think?* What do you, as the trainee, think about what happened? Can you identify any areas for change?
- *What Goal would you like to achieve?* What do you want to change? This can relate to the outcomes, rather than at this stage thinking about how you might achieve them.
- *Any Offers of how we should get there?* Do you have any ideas as to *how* to achieve your desired goal? Does your trainer, or any other group members, have any suggestions? Use the opportunity to rehearse suggestions.

An example of using the SET-GO approach might be following a consultation with an angry patient who has received a letter from the practice changing his medication from perindopril to ramipril.

- **See**: patient was very angry about the letter that he had received and continued to shout at the doctor throughout the consultation.
- **Else**: as the patient continued shouting he did not answer the questions that the doctor asked him about whether he had actually started the new medication.
- **Think**: being unable to defuse the patient's anger meant that the doctor was unable to move the consultation on and resolve the situation. The doctor did well in not responding to the patient's anger by getting angry himself.
- **Goal**: the doctor would like to be able to defuse angry patients effectively.
- **Offers**: perhaps letting angry patients talk until they run out of steam,* rather than interrupting them earlier in the consultation, or maybe acknowledging what you see: 'I can tell that you are very angry about this'. Practising these responses in a role play situation would be a good way of rehearsing this in preparation for your next angry patient.

UTILISING FEEDBACK EFFECTIVELY

Sometimes, however, regardless of how well the feedback is given we find it hard to make sense of. There is a tendency in all of us to develop one of two responses:

1. We accept the negative part of the feedback but try to explain it or justify it (or simply decide that the person who gave us the feedback is wrong and so we dismiss it entirely).
2. We focus on the positive and use it to reinforce what we already know to be true, rather than concentrating on areas for improvement.

The risk of both these responses is that the value of the feedback is lost, as is valuable time during which you could start to make positive change. For some OMGs this can mean failing their CSA, which could potentially have been avoided if they were ready to listen, and hear, what their GP training scheme had been saying to them for some time.

> I wish I had been able to take on board what my trainer had been saying earlier. As it was I just kept telling myself that he was wrong, that he didn't understand me. But then the CSA examiners agreed with him. Maybe for me I needed that shock to be ready to change, but I would hope others might learn from my experience.
>
> Abid

Phrase notes
* 'run out of steam' – to lose energy or become exhausted

By using a matrix to examine the feedback you can ensure that you get the maximum benefit from it for the future, and try to avoid falling into one of these traps.

	Positive	Negative
Expected		
Unexpected		

Feedback usually fits one of the categories in the matrix.

- **Positive/expected**: hopefully you will have a good idea of what you do well already, probably as a result of getting regular positive feedback! But rather than just hearing it and congratulating yourself, think about what you could do with this feedback. In particular, maybe you could think about how this particular strength might help you develop in other areas, or perhaps how you could use it to help develop others. Remembering this feedback can also really help your self-esteem when you feel that you are simply receiving constant criticism, or get some extreme negative feedback such as an exam failure.

- **Negative/expected**: again, often there are areas of our lives and work where we know that we need to make changes in order to improve. Perhaps you could try thinking about what strategies you have already tried in a particular area. Are they working? How could you make them more successful? Do you need any outside help to enable you to change? What would be the consequences of not changing?

- **Positive/unexpected**: this is a bit like a surprise birthday present and will hopefully give you a real lift. It is, however, then worth stepping back and thinking why you were surprised to hear it. Have you been dismissing this area of strength in your life? Why is that? How could you use it to develop further?

- **Negative/unexpected**: this is often the hardest feedback to accept and can evoke some pretty strong emotional reactions. You may need some time to take it on board,* but when you do, it can really help you in developing your self-awareness. You might need to think about other information that you need to be able to make sense of it, and perhaps check it out with other individuals. You might need some support to deal with the implications and some outside help in developing a plan to make small, achievable steps toward change. However, you might also find it helpful to reflect on how your life and work would improve if you are able to make such changes.

Phrase notes
* 'take it on board' – to understand and accept ideas and opinions which may affect the way that you behave in future

So, having received, and heard, the feedback that you have been given, how do you go about making changes? This is where the development of a personal development plan (PDP) is invaluable.

ACTION POINT 4

The next time you get feedback from your trainer, perhaps at your next tutorial, try fitting it into the feedback matrix. Are there any surprises? Try discussing these with your trainer.

YOUR PERSONAL DEVELOPMENT PLAN

Your PDP is your record of your learning or development needs along with a plan as to how you are intending to achieve it. During your GP training it may well be influenced by your learning log (indeed, you can export entries from the log directly into your PDP) but as you continue your professional development it may be refined to just four or five items each year that you review with your appraiser. One of the key points is that it is your *personal* development plan, which means that *your* PDP will probably look quite different from your colleagues' plans. So it is unlikely that a meaningful PDP will include mandatory requirements, such as passing your CSA, as they are applicable to everyone; although if this has been a particular challenge for you it would be entirely reasonable for it to appear as one of your PDP objectives.

The key to developing a good PDP is that the objectives that you put on it should be SMART. This is an acronym (with several variants) but which often stands for:

> **S** = specific
> **M** = measurable
> **A** = achievable
> **R** = relevant
> **T** = time-bound

Specific: this means that the objective is clear and unambiguous rather than a vague platitude. It often includes the 5 Ws:
1. *What*: what do I want to accomplish?
2. *Why*: specific reasons, purpose or benefits of the chosen goal.
3. *Who*: who is involved?
4. *Where*: identify a location.
5. *Which*: identify requirements and constraints.

Measurable: specifying criteria by which you can measure the goal helps to establish whether or not you are making progress in the right direction.

Sometimes this will be really concrete, such as passing an exam, or making a specific number of log entries. Other times it may be more reflective, such as improved consultation skills, and here, feedback may help you to work out whether you are en route to achieving your goal.

Achievable: setting a good objective may well stretch your current abilities but it should not be so extreme as to be completely unachievable. If it is, then it may be worth breaking it down into more manageable steps that help you to think about how you might achieve the desired outcome. For example, the first step in becoming the next chair of the RCGP might be to qualify as a fully fledged GP! Or, if that seems too simple, you might move up a level and make your goal that of getting elected to the RCGP council.

Relevant: working toward a relevant goal will help to motivate you and may also help you to gain support for your endeavours. For example, a GP registrar who wants to develop his or her consultation skills for general practice is likely to get more encouragement from his or her trainer than someone who wants to pass PACES (the specialty exams for hospital medicine) as, although worthwhile, this is not as immediately relevant to GPs and may, for some individuals, be a distraction from the areas that they need to concentrate on. (That is not to say that passing PACES is not an appropriate PDP objective, but it probably isn't for someone who has repeatedly failed his or her CSA.)

Time-bound: setting a completion date will help to ground your suggestions and give you a target to work toward.

So some examples of good PDP entries might be as follows.

Example 1

What is my development need?

I would like to improve my consultation skills particularly with more challenging patients, such as breaking bad news and substance misusers.

How do I plan to achieve it?

- To continue to practise my consulting in day-to-day practice and perhaps consider whether I can arrange to observe some sessions in the local prison with my trainer.
- Also to undertake some role plays with my peer group of GP trainees, looking particularly at more emotionally charged consultations, and exploring consulting models that are available for specific situations such as breaking bad news.

What evidence will I provide to show that I have attained it?

- Reflection in my e-portfolio, perhaps including teaching some of what I learn about consultation models to my GPStR colleagues.
- I will produce some videos of my consultations for discussion with my trainer.
- I will pass my CSA!

How will my practice improve as a result of this activity?

- I will be less like a rabbit in the headlights* with these consultations.
- Hopefully my timekeeping will also improve, as well as my ability to say 'no' appropriately.
- It may improve patient satisfaction but that might be adversely affected if I become more confident at declining inappropriate requests, such as diazepam for drug misusers.

Example 2

What is my development need?

I need to understand how general practice is funded in the UK.

How do I plan to achieve it?

- By discussing it with my trainer and a tutorial with the practice manager.
- Attend the annual accountants meeting.
- Review the changes to the Quality and Outcomes Framework (QOF) for 2013.

What evidence will I provide to show that I have achieved it?

- Reflection in my e-portfolio.
- Better opportunistic achievement of QOF indicators within routine consultations, perhaps an audit of a specific QOF area.

How will my practice improve as a result of this activity?

- I will have a greater understanding of what to look for when considering a future partnership.
- Improved practice income if I improve my ability to achieve QOF indicators.
- I will be more aware of prescribing and referral costs that may change these aspects of my practice.

Phrase notes
* 'rabbit in the headlights' – to be so frightened or surprised that you cannot move or think

> **ACTION POINT 5**
>
> Try to write a PDP objective that is personal to you and which is a SMART objective. Perhaps you could try using one of the ideas in this book as a starting point?

REFLECTIVE PRACTICE

All of the ideas above are focused on your ability to be a reflective practitioner, as they are about developing your critical appreciation of your practice. Recognising this can be really useful in helping to demystify the idea of reflective practice, which as a term can sometimes be difficult to comprehend. Developing reflection is one of the cornerstones of being a professional, as we can never get to the point where we can say that we know everything and have nothing left to learn. This can be at a knowledge level, or in relation to our skills and attitude. It is about recognising that competence is more than the accumulation of competencies. I (MF) remember being astonished when my trainer told me that selective serotonin reuptake inhibitors did not exist when he was at medical school and wondering how he got used to such a sea change* in practice. Yet even in our time in practice we can think of things that have changed significantly – for example, what the role of aspirin is in primary prevention of cardiovascular disease. We are also aware of the increasing complexity of practice and the patients who do not 'fit' neatly into predetermined boxes. This is increasingly the case as simpler protocol-driven endeavours are transferred to our colleagues, such as the growing network of nurse practitioners. Patients also continue to surprise us with their reactions to certain situations.

One of the key influences on professionalism in medicine has been not a medic but rather an architect, Donald Schön.[10] He talks about the fact that, as professionals, if we are to concentrate on the areas that are important to our patients, we need to be willing to inhabit the 'swampy lowlands' of practice, which are messy and confusing. He describes three fundamental constructs.

1. **Knowing in action (tacit or unspoken knowledge)**: this is our unconscious competence, the way in which we instinctively know how to do something. For example, we hope that by the time you reach your GP training there are certain fundamental skills that you can do easily, such as taking blood, that are nonetheless unfamiliar to the average bystander.
2. **Reflection in action (thinking on your feet)**: this is reflection that occurs at a time when you can still make a difference to the particular event in practice – 'on the spot' reflection. For example, you might notice that the patient

---

Phrase notes
* 'sea change' – a significant transformation

whose blood you have been taking suddenly turns pale and looks like she is about to faint, so you get her to lie down.

3. **Reflection on action (retrospective thinking)**: this is what you do after the event, in order to make sense of how using your knowledge in practice and reflection in practice resulted in the observed outcome. For example, you might conclude that there are things that you could have done differently, such as ask the patient if she has ever felt faint before when someone has been taking her blood, and, if so, consider getting her to lie down before starting. Or perhaps you might find something that helps explain why this particular patient reacted differently (such as her not having had any breakfast!) compared with other patients from whom you have taken blood.

Obviously the example we have given of taking blood from someone is a very simple one, designed just to help illustrate what Schön means by his two types of reflection. Yet, reflective practice really comes into its own when we think about more complex situations.

Gawande,[11] a surgical resident in the United States, says:

> We look for medicine to be an orderly field of knowledge and procedure. But it is not. It is an imperfect science, an enterprise of constantly changing knowledge, uncertain information, fallible individuals, and at the same time lives on the line. There is science in what we do, yes, but also habit, intuition, and sometimes plain old guessing. The gap between what we know and what we aim for persists. And this gap complicates everything we do.

Recognising that this 'gap' exists for everyone can be very liberating, but it can also be a particular challenge for OMGs who are sometimes used to a culture where the doctor is expected to know everything.

> Back home, in Iraq, you are expected to know everything. Realising that there was another way, that I didn't have to do that made a huge difference. Of course there are some things that you do have to know but often you just need to know how to find something you don't know, to recognise when you don't know the answer, which is a skill in itself, I guess.
>
> Arrass

So where do you start if you want to develop your skills as a reflective practitioner? The obvious answer would be with your patients, who are one of the richest sources of learning material available to you.

LEARNING FROM PATIENTS

Gibbs's[12] reflective cycle (*see* Figure 2.5) can be a helpful tool in getting you to start to think about how you might learn from a particular situation.

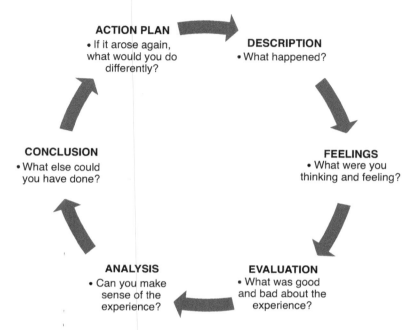

FIGURE 2.5 Gibbs's reflective cycle

Sometimes it helps to understand something if you can see an example of it being used. So here is one of our reflections on a recent patient encounter, using Gibbs's reflective cycle, which would also make a really good learning log entry!

Description (what happened?)

A 16-year-old girl came to see me on Wednesday requesting post-coital contraception (PCC). The previous weekend she had unprotected sexual intercourse and had gone to the chemist for the morning-after pill. The chemist told her it would cost over £25 and as she didn't have the money to pay she left without it.

Feelings (what were you thinking and feeling?)

I was angry on the girl's behalf that the chemist had turned her away without helping her to find another way of accessing care. I was also frustrated that the girl had taken until Wednesday to choose to consult again.

Evaluation (what was good and bad about the experience?)

I was able to give the girl EllaOne and offer her a coil, which she declined. I also advised her about accessing PCC if the situation arose again, as well as address her ongoing need for contraception. I also think and hope that I made her consultation a positive experience, such that she would consult again if she were in a similar situation.

Analysis (can you make sense of the experience?)

I tried to work out, sensitively, why there was such a delay in her presenting and I think it was because she (a) was embarrassed and (b) didn't realise that I might still be able to help her.

Conclusion (what else could you have done?)

I could (and probably should) have gone back to the original chemist and challenged them, as they could have signposted her to other places that she could access care, such as out of hours (OOH) or the minor injuries unit.

Action plan (if it arose again, what would you do differently?)

I will make sure that everyone who comes for regular contraception knows how to access post-coital contraception, particularly at the weekend. I will talk to the partners about putting some posters up in the waiting room. I will also find out about whether chemists can offer PCC free of charge.

ACTION POINT 6

Complete a Gibbs's reflective cycle for a recent patient encounter. What learning needs did it help you identify?

Another way of learning from patients might be by keeping a log (which can take a number of physical forms, and doesn't have to be written) of times when you identify areas that you want to look into further. The idea is to note down the area that you want to address as soon as it occurs, even during a consultation, so as to be able to come back to it later.

Areas that you might want to look at are:

- gaps in your clinical knowledge (e.g. the latest hypertension guidelines)
- skills that you would like to acquire for the future (e.g. joint injections)
- difficulties that arose within the consultation (e.g. being able to defuse an angry patient).

I tried keeping a log of when I came across something I didn't know. It really helped me, as I discovered that I was really uncomfortable with women's health issues so I arranged a tutorial on this with one of the female partners.

Daniel

These are often referred to as **PUNs and DENs**,[13] where the patients' unmet needs (PUNs) help identify doctors' educational needs (DENs).

ACTION POINT 7

Keep a learning log (in whatever form you like) for a week of patients' unmet needs. Try to record them as they occur, within the consultation or between patients. Review the list at the end of the week (if not before) and then spend some time addressing the learning needs that you have identified.

Hopefully this chapter has given you a number of suggestions to help you learn how to learn. We expect you will find some of them useful and some of them will make no sense to you at all. Unfortunately, there is no magic answer, no alternative to putting in the hard work. Although we hope that you will at least start to recognise that you can never know everything and that this is not your fault!

REFERENCES

1. Maslow AH. A theory of human motivation. *Psychol Rev.* 1943; **50**(4): 370–96.
2. General Medical Council (GMC). *Good Medical Practice*. London: GMC; 2013. Available at: www.gmc-uk.org/guidance/ethical_guidance/11817.asp (accessed 2 May 2013).
3. Fleming ND. I'm different; not dumb. Modes of presentation (VARK) in the tertiary classroom. In: Zelmer A, editor. *Research Development in Higher Education, Proceedings of the 1995 Annual Conference of the Higher Education and Research Development Society of Australasia (HERDSA)*. Volume 18. Sydney: HERDSA; 1995; pp. 308–13.
4. Honey P, Mumford A. *The Manual of Learning Styles*. Maidenhead, UK: Peter Honey Publications; 1982.
5. Kolb D. *Experiential Learning: experience as the source of learning development*. Englewood Cliffs, NJ: Prentice Hall; 1984.
6. Gardner H. *Frames of Mind: theory of multiple intelligences*. New York, NY: Basic Books; 1983.
7. Luft J, Ingham H. The Johari window, a graphic model of interpersonal awareness. *Proceedings of the Western Training Laboratory in Group Development*. Los Angeles, CA: UCLA; 1955.
8. Pendleton D, Schofield D, Tate P, *et al. The New Consultation: developing doctor-patient communication*. Oxford: Oxford University Press; 2003.
9. Silverman J, Draper J, Kurtz SM. The Calgary-Cambridge approach to communication skills teaching: the SET-GO method of descriptive feedback. *Educ Gen Pract.* 1997; **8**: 16–23.
10. Schön DA. *The Reflective Practitioner: how professionals think in action*. Aldershot: Basic Books; 1983.

11. Gawande A. *Complications: a surgeon's notes on an imperfect science*. London: Profile Books; 2002.

12. Gibbs G. *Learning by Doing: a guide to teaching and learning methods*. Oxford: Further Education Unit, Oxford Polytechnic; 1988.

13. Eve R. *PUNs and DENs: discovering learning needs in general practice*. Oxford: Radcliffe Publishing; 2003.

CHAPTER 3

Consulting as a general practitioner

Learning how to consult as a GP is very different from what you may have been used to in hospital practice, particularly if you have only worked in a hospital setting as a relatively junior practitioner. GPs are still part of a wider team, particularly with initiatives such as clinical commissioning groups and peer review of referrals. However, on a daily basis, consulting as a GP involves a very small partnership: that of you and the patient in front of you. In most instances (particularly when you are fully qualified) it will be up to you to formulate a shared, agreed management plan with your patient without needing to consult anyone else. There will, of course, still be instances when you need to seek advice from either your hospital or practice colleagues, but one of the key skills that you need to master as a GP is that of being able to deal with uncertainty.

Yet with this responsibility also comes a degree of independence and flexibility. Particularly if you are a partner, rather than a salaried employee, you will have the freedom to influence the services on offer from your practice, such that they really meet your practice population's needs. Clearly you will not be able to afford unlimited initiatives but you will be able to decide whether, for example, offering counselling free of charge is something that you would be interested in, or whether you would prefer to offer a youth drop-in service.

The time pressures on consulting are also very different in general practice. The usual consultation length is 10 minutes, although there is sometimes the flexibility to book longer appointments when needed. Indeed, some practices have been experimenting with allowing patients to decide how long an appointment they need, with times varying from 5 to 20 minutes. This might seem like an incredibly short time for any meaningful intervention. However, it would not be uncommon for a GP to be involved with the same practice for over 30 years. John Launer[1] describes this as being able to provide 'ultra-brief, ultra-long therapy'. Such long-term involvement provides us with the huge privilege of being involved in our patients' lives; sharing in the important milestones of birth, serious illness and death. Being curious about our patients' lives, and seeing them as people rather than simply 'disease carriers', is a key part of learning to consult effectively. For example, working out how Mr Smith is related to Mrs Jones can make a huge difference to understanding her abdominal pain. Knowing what makes someone tick* can be crucial in helping to motivate him or her to change.

This level of continuity of care is one of the cornerstones of UK general practice. Admittedly, initiatives such as advanced access have made it more likely that a patient may end up consulting a number of different doctors. However, these are still likely to be individuals within the same practice organisation, and thus sharing access to the entire patient record. Unlike in many other countries, the GP is the first port of call[†] regardless of the presenting symptoms, and patients cannot shop around[‡] between different practices depending on what they perceive their need to be at any one time. In order to access specialist care the patient first has to present to his or her GP. This means that we are well placed to think holistically about what is best for the patient as a person rather than simply focusing on disease processes. It helps us to recognise that while disease is the cause of sickness, illness is the unique experience of that sickness and may vary significantly between different individuals. However, it also presents the challenge of keeping up to date across a wide spectrum of disciplines. For the health system this 'gatekeeper role' is also a way of controlling spiralling health costs, as well as maintaining a bird's-eye view[§] as to how different diseases and, perhaps more important, their treatments, influence one another.

It also means that we have unrivalled opportunities to promote health within our practice population. We can be proactive in encouraging individuals to take more responsibility for their own health rather than simply reacting to any symptoms that they develop. By influencing individuals we can also influence wider public health issues, which will have significant impact for the future. Practices have been responsible for initiatives such as walking groups and even cooking classes for healthy eating, if this is what they identify as priorities for their particular patient population. This is in addition to the more conventional medical interventions for health promotion such as smoking cessation groups.

Finally, it is worth remembering that the NHS offers treatment that is free at the point of delivery to an individual patient. The only obvious exception

---

Phrase notes

* 'makes someone tick' – something that motivates someone or that makes someone behave in a certain way
† 'first port of call' – the first place you stop to do something
‡ 'shop around' – visit different establishments to compare them (usually on the basis of price and quality) before deciding where to get a particular service or item
§ 'bird's-eye view' – a view seen from high above

to this is prescription charges, which are directly paid by the patient in some parts of the UK. This means that there is no financial incentive for doctors to repeatedly call their patients back. It also means that no patient should be precluded from medical care because of poverty or multiple medical conditions. Admittedly, it does bring with it the inevitable challenge of waiting lists and some rationing of care, but these issues are common to most developed countries' healthcare systems, to a greater or lesser extent. Sometimes patients who are complaining about aspects of NHS care are surprised when you share with them the actual cost of their monthly prescription!

This means that UK general practice may well be very different from how family practice is approached in your home country. In the UK, general practice has been a recognised specialty for many years, during which time it has been continually refined. In contrast in many other countries it is more of an emerging specialty and so at an earlier stage of development. This does not mean that our system is better; indeed, it probably isn't in at least some respects but it does mean that it has developed its own culture and practice. Given that you are training to work in this system it is important that you try to make sense of this culture, not least because it is what patients have come to expect.

> The culture difference has a major impact on consultations. Where I graduated from people usually prefer to be reassured in all conditions that they will get better even if they are in end stage. If you don't give them a hope and medications 'even if tonics', they won't believe in you and seek advice from others. They have a high hope in God and that a miracle will happen. Patients generally have high respect for doctors and they are grateful even if things go wrong.
>
> Giving options and sharing the treatment decision with the patient is almost absent and it is up to the doctor to choose what they think is the best option for the patient and patients will always respect that.
>
> Abi

> Back in Africa, after graduation you aspire to be a hospital consultant. GPs are unknown.
>
> Gloria

ACTION POINT 1

Take a moment to think about how UK general practice compares with that of your home country. Try remembering a specific patient with multiple medical problems – in what ways do they get better care in the UK? In what ways would the care in your home country be preferable from this patient's perspective?

NAVIGATING THE CONSULTATION

Having thought about some of the wider picture let's now move on to think about how to maximise the benefit of a particular consultation. Inevitably, some of the themes discussed here will be echoed in other chapters, particularly the ones on communication skills and succeeding in assessment. This is because consulting is really just one of the many ways in which we communicate with patients, and the MRCGP exam, particularly the CSA component, is designed to test that ability. Thinking about consulting as an extension of communication skills can be really helpful in demystifying what may not actually be such a difficult skill to master.

A good place to start would be thinking about how you find your way, or navigate, through the consultation. This can be particularly helpful for people who struggle with keeping time, as that is often because of looping back and forward between different aspects of the consultation. Essentially, a good consultation will involve you finding out why the patient has come and, only once you have done this, then moving onto the management of the problem. This is sometimes described as 'the consultation bridge',[2] as you only cross over to management once you have got sufficient information to inform your decision-making.

Finding out why a patient has come is, of course, not quite as simple as it might sound! It includes the details of the patient's symptoms, how this is affecting the patient's life, what the patient's health beliefs are about the situation and the results of any investigations and examination (both physical and mental). It also involves checking with the patient (of which more later) that *you* have understood the information that they have shared with you. Finally, it may also include some medical detective work to try to exclude red flags or narrow down the range of potential differential diagnoses. Interestingly, this narrowing of the possible outcomes can actually involve broadening out the patient's perspective as you encourage them to think about the presence of symptoms that they may never have attributed to their presenting complaint. Navigating this terrain skilfully is what separates a competent medical practitioner from an interested party, such as a friend or relative, who may be equally competent at active listening and eliciting the patient's concerns but who will not have the medical background to put what they hear into context.

Once you have established this, then, and only then, can you move into discussing management options. This involves linking your explanation back to the patient's reason for coming and explaining the possible management plans. Then, in sharing this management plan you need to give the patient enough information about the various options for him or her to be able to make an informed decision as to which one to choose. It involves taking into account the patient's preferences for a particular management strategy, the likelihood of success of any given strategy and considering any contraindications such as drug allergies. Finally, you will need to check with the patient that *he or she* have

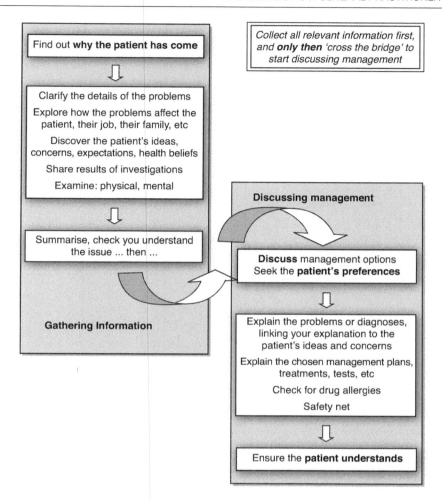

FIGURE 3.1 The consultation bridge. Reproduced with the kind permission of Damian Kenny, www.damiankenny.co.uk, from Kenny D. A consultation navigation tool. *Education for Primary Care.* 2012; **23**(1): 41.

understood *you*! Being open to the idea that a patient may not have understood you when you feel that you have done a perfect job of explaining something to them can be quite threatening for some people, and may be something that you find that you have to work on. For some OMGs, a patient's lack of understanding can feed into a whole belief system about their ability (or lack of) to use English appropriately, or that they will never be accepted by English patients. If this is you, then you may need to do some work thinking about how you respond in such situations, for while inevitably there probably are some patients who are racist, these are undoubtedly the minority. All of us are misunderstood by patients some of the time, perhaps because we are having a bad day or perhaps because they are. Tailoring your explanations to suit particular patients is a real skill, so practising it certainly helps, but so does not making assumptions about how to approach it with a particular patient because of his or her background. We are all unique individuals as doctors, and our patients are unique individuals too – one size certainly doesn't fit all.*

ACTION POINT 2

- Watch a video of one of your consultations. Make a note of the phrases you use and then grade them as either I (information) or M (management). Now draw a graph of how often you loop between the two parts of the consultation.
- Now observe someone who you consider to be a good consulter (e.g. your trainer) in a joint surgery. Again initially record the phrases as you hear them, and then go back and grade them as I or M. How does this person's graph compare with yours?

It is probably worth looking at more than one of your consultations using the consultation bridge tool to see if there are particular types of consultation that you struggle with. For example, some people struggle with those that include a formal examination component, by tending to leave this late in the consultation and then having to revisit their ideas around potential diagnoses and management due to unexpected findings. For other people it is consultations where there is not a clear presenting complaint that are more of an issue, or cases where you have to try to remain patient focused in follow-up consultations when the patient has been asked to come back for his or her results. Or perhaps for you it is the consultation where there seems to be only one right answer, such as in an emergency situation, where sharing management options and valuing the patient's contribution is more of a challenge.

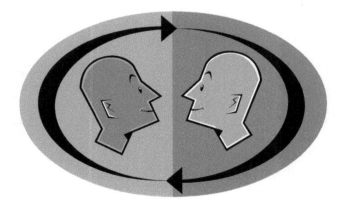

Phrase notes

* 'one size fits all (or doesn't fit all)' – the idea that the same approach or product can be used in every instance

CONSULTATION MODELS

Using consultation models can be another way of thinking about how to develop your consultation skills; however, these are not a magic answer to being an effective consulter (or to succeeding at postgraduate assessment). Rather, they are signposts that can help you on the way. If you talk to any experienced GP you will probably find that he or she does not follow any particular recognised formal model. Instead, the GP will have taken parts of each model that he or she has found useful and adapted it to suit his or her own style and personality. The GP may return to thinking about a model sometimes, such as when he or she gets stuck with a particular patient and does not know how to move things on. Usually, however, the GP's use of models will be invisible and unconscious, like looking in the rear-view mirror becomes once you pass your driving test.

SOMETHING TO THINK ABOUT

Consulting is complex, not complicated! You cannot follow a consultation model rigidly and expect a perfect outcome – it is not about following a recipe to make the perfect cake!

So if consultation models are not the magic answer, how do they help? Let's start by considering what some of the common consultation models offer. Most of the commonly used models fall into three types.

1. **Task-based**: these models tell you what to do. Examples would include Neighbour,[3] Pendleton *et al.*[4] and Stott and Davis.[5] Being able to apply these models well can be a challenge for those who qualified abroad, as these are the models that can be most likened to a recipe. Sometimes OMGs get frustrated when they feel that they have followed all these tasks and still not got a good outcome. The skill comes from knowing how to apply the model, and how to respond to the patient's contribution such that it becomes an interaction between two people. This is what makes consulting fluent, when the patient's response to a particular question informs the next question, rather than the doctor rigidly following a list of rote questions.

2. **Descriptive**: these models are based on watching doctors and patients and seeing what they do. Examples would include Tuckett *et al.*[6] and Byrne and Long.[7] These can be really useful tools for looking at some of your own consultations. Where they are really helpful is looking at where the consultation appeared to go off-track. Sometimes by watching repeated videos you can identify, for example, that whenever you ask a patient a particular question he or she responds in a particular way. Being able to look back at consultations where you have changed your approach can be really helpful in enabling you to determine what works well for the future. Although it is,

of course, worth remembering that not all patients will respond in the same way to a similar enquiry, nor, indeed, will the same patient always respond in the same way to the same enquiry asked at different times.

3. **Explanatory**: these models seek to explore *why* doctors and patients behave in particular ways. Examples would include Helman,[8] Berne[9] and Balint.[10] Again these can be more useful for OMGs as they move beyond the application of tasks to trying to gain some background understanding as to why a consultation has gone in a particular direction, or why a patient has tried a particular treatment or failed to agree with your plan of treatment. This can be a step on from the simple descriptive models, as it can help to explain why some patients will respond differently to what appears, at face value,* to be a very similar question.

The apparent simplicity of task-based consultation models can be attractive to those in training, particularly if you are struggling with consulting. However, using repeated observations to look at *what* actually happened and using these as a springboard to think about *why* it happened can be incredibly useful in helping you to identify areas that need to change. That is why the use of video consultations remains a key part of GP training despite not being an essential part of the assessment process anymore.

The following sections of this chapter look briefly at some of the common consultation models, including some of the pitfalls that can accompany using them too rigorously. If any of them particularly catch your eye[†] then you can read about them in more detail in the source texts, which are detailed in the chapter references.

McWhinney's consultation model[11]

Even while you were in junior hospital positions you probably unconsciously used a consultation model that was embedded in your medical training, the so-called medical model. This concentrates on the doctor's perspective on the consultation, using history and examination to formulate a diagnosis and appropriate clinical management plan that will sort out the problem, but not necessarily the patient. In contrast to this, McWhinney's model (*see* Figure 3.2) seeks to draw together both the doctor's and the patient's agendas. It uses the concept of a disease framework for the medical aspects and counterbalances this with the illness framework, which highlights the issues for the particular patient. Familiarising yourself with this model can therefore be a good bridging step before launching into some of the other consultation models that can seem much further removed from what you are used to.

Phrase notes

* 'face value' – to accept someone or something just as it appears; to believe that the way things appear is the way they really are

† 'catch your eye' – attract your interest

McWhinney's model introduces the idea that patients are more than disease carriers. The underlying medical problem is the disease, and the patient's experience of that disease is the patient's illness. It recognises the idea that patients can be ill without having any disease – the 'tired all the time' patient being a classic example of this. The converse is also true in that the patient can have a disease without being ill, such as the patient with hyperlipidaemia. It is the doctor's job to bring together these two aspects of the consultation, the biomedical approach *and* how this particular patient is experiencing this situation.

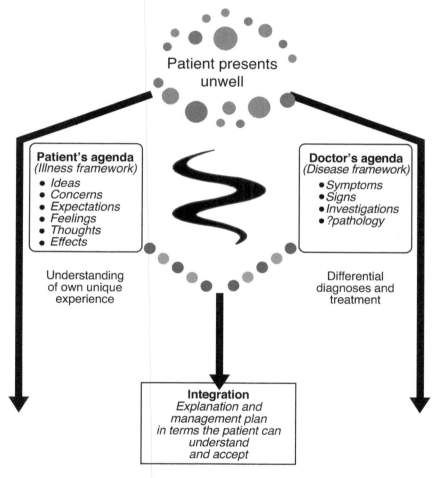

FIGURE 3.2 McWhinney's consultation model

Neighbour[3]

Roger Neighbour is a GP who has devised a consultation model that is now familiar to most GP registrars. He refers to this consultation model as being like a journey, with waypoints signposting the direction of travel. You may find it a really useful consultation model for OMGs, as it involves a broad-brush approach, which makes it less susceptible to the recipe problem! Some people find his book a challenge; if this is you then that is fine, but just make sure that you don't throw the baby out with the bathwater* and perhaps explore one of the summary texts of his approach.

Neighbour's model has five key tasks, or skills.

1. **Connecting**: this involves listening to what the patient is saying, demonstrating empathy and reaching a joint understanding of what the problem and possible solutions are. It includes simple actions like welcoming the patient and introducing yourself but also the subtleties of your body language and non-verbal communication. Connecting is not solely restricted to the beginning of a consultation, although obviously starting off well is important. You can continue to connect with patients as you progress – for example, by using the words and language that they have used when summarising or handing over.

2. **Summarising**: this is about feeding back to the patient what you have heard, which gives him or her a chance to point out any misunderstandings or things that you have missed – this is your opportunity to show how well you have connected. A good summary will not only include the basic history that you have obtained from the patient but also link back to what you have found out about the patient's ideas, concerns and expectations. A good summary can really help to focus the second part of a consultation and ensure that you have really got to the crux of the issues, both medically and from the patient's viewpoint. However, it is important to use this fluently rather than slavishly applying it to *all* your consultations, as there are clearly times when it will be less appropriate. Sometimes an effective summary can also be a good way of 'pressing the pause button' in an emotionally charged consultation and may help, for example, to defuse a patient's anger.

3. **Handing over**: this is about sharing the responsibility and the management plan, being 'patient-centred' – this is where you need to give the patient enough information that he or she can be engaged in a meaningful way in the management rather than simply telling the patient what to do. How much you can hand over responsibility to the patient varies depending on the clinical scenario. For example, it might be appropriate to be more doctor centred with a patient presenting with cardiac-sounding chest pain or other serious symptoms, particularly if the patients themselves do not recognise the severity of their condition. However, there is usually scope to demonstrate elements of patient centred-ness even in this type of consultation. Tailoring how much choice you give a patient to his or her level of

---

Phrase notes

* 'throw the baby out with the bathwater' – to discard something valuable with something that is not desired, usually unintentionally

understanding and the seriousness of his or her underlying complaint can be a really effective way of being patient centred.

4. **Safety-netting**: this is about ensuring that you have enough information to make the right decision, such as asking about 'red flags' that may not be apparent to the patient *and* ensuring that the patient has enough information to know when, and how, to seek help appropriately should the situation change. This might include, for example, information about the local OOH service or even when to call an emergency ambulance.
5. **Housekeeping**: this is about stopping, reflecting and being able to put one patient aside so that you can be fully available to the next one. This could include making sure your notes are written up, any referrals done or at least noted for later. However, it is also a good excuse (should you need one) for a cup of tea!

In order to effectively use Neighbour's model it is worth thinking about your ability to listen and to summarise what you have heard.

ACTION POINT 3

How good a listener are you? Try recording a feature on the radio or downloading an interesting podcast. Listen to it for a couple of minutes then try summarising it to a friend or colleague (or writing down a short summary). Then listen again – how does your summary compare? What did you miss?

Cambridge–Calgary model[12]

Cambridge–Calgary is also a useful model, as this is the one that is most closely aligned with the CSA. Thinking about it broadly there are six main themes:
1. Initiating the session
2. Gathering information
3. Providing structure
4. Building relationship
5. Explanation and planning
6. Closing the session.

These are, however, broken down into lots of smaller, discrete units, with a total of over 70 micro-skills that are described. For example, in initiating the session there are elements designed to help achieve initial rapport, such as introducing yourself and attending to the patient's comfort. This then moves onto discussing the reason for the patient's attendance. These small subsections can be incredibly useful in focusing your attention on the areas of the consultation that you need to develop. There is a very real risk, however, that some OMGs follow the list religiously and are then frustrated to find that the consultation still doesn't go as well as they had hoped initially. This is most likely to happen when you don't allow the earlier parts of the consultation to inform the latter aspects and insist on asking the patient questions to which they have already volunteered an answer.

An example of this would be as follows.

Patient: I've come to see you about my headache …
Doctor: Tell me some more about your headache.
Patient: Well, it's really bad. It stops me concentrating on my revision and I'm really worried it's something serious like a brain tumour.
Doctor: Are you worried about it being something serious? [*Here you are completely ignoring the fact that the patient has already disclosed concerns regarding a possible brain tumour.*]

A much better response would be as follows.

Doctor: Why are you worried it might be a brain tumour? [*This acknowledges the patient's contribution to the consultation, so demonstrating that you were actually listening and also enabling the consultation to move on.*]

You could also move this same consultation on by asking the following (probably after addressing the patient's concerns about a potential brain tumour, as this may well stop the patient concentrating on anything else you might say).

Doctor: Does it affect you in any other way than stopping you revising?

Or even the following, using the patient's cue to set the problem into context for this particular patient.

Doctor: You mentioned you are having difficulty revising. What exams are you studying for? [*Patient gives name of exams.*] Are you worrying about them?

One of the most useful parts of Cambridge–Calgary, however, is the section that describes explanation and planning. In particular, there are aspects that relate to providing the patient with the correct amount and type of information, which introduces the idea of 'chunks and checks'. What this means is that the GP divides the information that he or she would like to share with the patient into manageable amounts (the 'chunks'), then checks that the patient has understood this, and uses the patient's response as a guide as to how to proceed. Regularly checking how much the patient understands can be useful in determining how much to break down the information into manageable chunks. This will obviously vary depending upon the complexity of the information that you are trying to convey as well as the patient's intellectual ability and any previous discussions that the patient may have had with you, or another practitioner or friend. Taking note of how the patient has given you information in the first part of a consultation can be helpful in guiding you as to how quickly he or she can absorb information.

An example of this might be the teenager who comes in to discuss how to manage her period pains. Rather than listing a long list of potential options, you could break this down into the two main focuses of potential treatment; namely, either treating the pain when it occurs or using hormonal manipulation to switch off the natural cycle. You would, however, need to give sufficient information about these two potential classes of treatment, rather than simply listing them, for the patient to be able to make an informed choice. Depending upon how the patient responded, you would then go into further detail of the option she wanted to explore further – for example, breaking down the hormonal option still further to combined oral contraceptive pill, implant, progesterone injection or intrauterine system. This means that you are targeting the information that you give to how the patient responds and that the patient is informed enough to make a sensible choice.

ACTION POINT 4

Get together with some colleagues and brainstorm how you might subdivide other treatment options.

Examples include:

- *acne* – topical treatments, hormonal treatments, antibiotics
- *atrial fibrillation* – rate control, rhythm control, anticoagulation
- *menopausal symptoms* – patient information, hormone replacement therapy, specific symptom control, complementary therapies
- *contraception* – hormonal versus non-hormonal or oral versus non-oral
- *depression* – talking therapies, antidepressant medication, social input or watchful waiting
- *back pain* – painkillers, physical treatments (osteopathy and chiropractor) or physiotherapy, onward referral for investigation and treatment.

It is worth remembering that patients often find it hard to admit that they don't understand what you have said. If you just ask them 'is that clear?' or similar then you are likely to get an automatic 'yes' as your response. So it can be useful to think about how you might check that a patient has understood you. Sometimes placing the potential blame for any misunderstanding onto the quality of your explanation can be useful, such as:

I realise I've gone through a lot of things and it may be that I haven't made them all clear. Which bits do I need to run through again?

Checking understanding can, however, be one of the areas where OMGs may resort to inappropriate rote questioning. You will find more information on this in Chapter 4 on communication skills. If a patient tells you that his wife sent him to see you, then it may well be that asking him what he would tell his wife when he gets home is an appropriate question. You could even link it back to his opening statement:

> You mentioned that your wife had persuaded you to come and see me. I was wondering what you might tell her about what we've discussed?

However, for other patients this question might be completely inappropriate. So the skill of consulting comes not only from having a variety of phrases and questions that you can use but, just as importantly, knowing *when* to say *what*. For example, I (MF) can certainly tell you that if you were to ask my mother what she was going tell my father when she got home it would not be well received (although they are happily married)! Instead, you would have to find an alternative way of checking that she had understood what you had tried to explain.

Pendleton *et al.*[4]

This is the model on which the consultation observation tool (part of the WPBA component of the MRCGP exam) is based, so it may well be worth looking into further. It is again a task-based system that has seven main tasks.
1. To **define the reason** for the patient's attendance, including:
   a. the nature and history of the problems
   b. their aetiology
   c. the patient's ideas, concerns and expectations
   d. the effects of the problems
2. To consider **other problems**:
   a. continuing problems
   b. at-risk factors
3. With the patient, to choose an **appropriate action** for each problem
4. To achieve a **shared understanding** of the problems with the patient
5. To **involve the patient** in the management and encourage them to accept appropriate responsibility
6. To **use time and resources** appropriately (a) in the consultation (b) in the long term
7. To establish or maintain a **relationship** with the patient that makes it easier for the other tasks to be achieved.

Although this model looks like it should work well, with a logical sequence, we are sure you will have realised by now that unfortunately not all consultations follow such a good order. So there is a degree of skill, as with all models, in being able to use this framework. It does, however, put a sound emphasis on gaining the patient's perspective as well as trying to work out where the patient is coming from. Sometimes it helps to get rid of the potential jargon element of ideas, concerns and expectations. Instead, try to find out what the patient's **thoughts** are about the problem, any **worries** the patient may have about either its cause or its effect on his or her life, and, finally, what the patient **hopes** you might be able to do to help him or her address it.

As always, don't push things too far! Some patients may indeed have obscure health beliefs that you will not get to unless you ask them directly, as you have no knowledge of the background of their lives. For example, I (MF) remember a patient who was concerned that a flu-like illness was really Weil's disease, as the patient had fallen into a lock on a canal boat trip 2 weeks previously. There is no way that anyone would have been able to find that out without directly asking. However, we have had other patients who have genuinely not thought about what might be causing their symptoms and who, while they don't mind being asked once, start feeling interrogated when the doctor repeatedly quizzes them about what they think is going on. Being truly patient centred means being able to recognise and adapt to patients who prefer a more paternalistic approach to some aspects of the consultation, while still empowering them with their decision-making around their management plans.

> Sometimes patients do come with ideas about their condition, but not always. I think the idea of a hidden agenda is too emphasised sometimes. So as IMGs we struggle to know how far to push.
>
> Katya

ACTION POINT 5

- During the next week make a list of the patients you see and what their thoughts, worries and hopes have been about their problems.
- Also make a note of how you established this – did you have to ask them directly or did they volunteer the information to you? Did you find any particularly helpful phrases in this regard?

Balint[10]

Michael Balint, the son of a GP, described a number of ideas and philosophies that can really aid our understanding of consultations, particularly with patients with whom we have a longer-term relationship but with whom we are struggling to make progress. He does not describe a consultation model so much as another way of approaching the consultation altogether. This is a completely different way of thinking about consultations compared with what you will probably be used to in a hospital environment, except perhaps in mental health settings. Balint maintained that the psychological, physical and social aspects of a consultation could not be separated from one another, as they always coexist. After all, we all know that psychological problems can manifest with physical symptoms (think of anxiety leading to palpitations and irritable bowel syndrome), and organic disease can certainly have psychological consequences. Balint believed that the ability to be able to explore all these aspects of the doctor–patient relationship simply required developing the appropriate skills, rather than being dependent on the doctor's personality.

Some of Balint's ideas have now become very well known, in particular the idea of an 'entry ticket' and 'the hidden agenda'. These ideas suggest that sometimes patients present with a simple problem as a way of testing out what they think of the doctor, before deciding whether to disclose the real reason for their attendance. Bearing in mind that a patient may have a hidden agenda is an important skill, as otherwise you may miss the real point of the consultation. However, it is entirely possible to swing too far in the other direction and assume that every patient has a hidden agenda and that it is just a matter of determining what it is. This can lead to patients having a feeling of being interrogated, such as when they are repeatedly asked about their ideas, concerns and expectations. The key skill is being able to balance being attentive and approachable enough, picking up on cues, so that patients are able to disclose difficult or embarrassing things to you, with not appearing to chastise patients who have genuinely chosen to consult with a minor issue. This can be more difficult than it sounds!

The idea of what to pick up on in a consultation is another aspect of consulting that Balint touches on, with the phrases 'selective attention' and 'selective neglect'. This refers to the idea that we sometimes choose to neglect certain aspects of the consultation, and place constraints on what it is acceptable to explore in a given situation. This means that we may recognise the cue but choose not to pursue it, thus changing the consultation into one that is much more doctor centred. This could be for a number of different reasons: some practical, such as the need to finish on time in order to collect your children from nursery; some emotional, such as a situation having too much resonance for us to be able to deal with it or anxiety that we will open the proverbial 'Pandora's box'* and not know what to do with the contents. All of us will do this at some points in our career, but it is probably best not to do it within the context of your CSA! It is also worth stopping and thinking about this at times of major stress or personal challenge, as we cannot predict what problems a patient will bring to the consulting room. For example, if you have

---

Phrase notes

* 'Pandora's box' – a source of unforeseen and extensive troubles: based on the Greek mythology of a box that Zeus gave to Pandora with instructions that she not open it; she gave in to her curiosity and opened it and all the miseries and evils flew out to afflict mankind

been recently bereaved it may be that you need to take some time out before returning to work in order to be able to fully offer yourself to patients facing similar situations.

This is because offering ourselves, to at least some extent, is an essential component of many consultations. This has an incredibly therapeutic effect for some patients, what Balint described as the 'doctor as a drug'. This can be particularly pertinent in certain situations, such as mental health or palliative care scenarios with carers, when we may feel that we have nothing to offer. What we really mean is that we cannot fix the patient's situation; however, we can sit with the patient in his or her distress. In these situations being particularly aware of our own feelings can be especially important in influencing patients. We also need to recognise that, as with any drug, some patients may become dependent on us as 'a drug' and this has significant consequences for our workload and the rationing of our time, which, just like any other asset, has limits.

It is in these more emotionally challenging situations that another of Balint's key ideas can be important, the idea of the 'flash'. This refers to that moment when suddenly it all seems to make sense! When it happens it is incredibly satisfying and really helps to move things forward with what are often very challenging, potentially 'heartsink' patients. In our experience it has happened most often when we have been able to identify a number of jigsaw pieces that we can finally put together to make a recognisable, often beautiful, picture. The pieces might include the symptoms the patient brings to the consultation and the feelings that they provoke in us, but also perhaps working out something else such as a family relationship that we had not previously identified or exploring why they always consult on the same day. An example might be my (MF) old primary school teacher who always consulted me (in a practice without personal lists) and who would then start each consultation with the phrase 'this is so embarrassing ...' I could never understand why he chose to consult me until one day when, unusually, his wife came with him and mentioned how great it was to see what one of his pupils had achieved. It turned out that seeing me reminded him that, even though he had been forced into early retirement on mental health grounds, and not entirely voluntarily, seeing one of his ex-pupils having achieved the status of being a well-respected GP made him feel much less of a failure; a fact that he was able to hang onto when he was feeling particularly low.

ACTION POINT 6

Over the next week, think about the consultations that occur that don't seem to make sense. Are there any aspects of Balint's work that you can apply to these situations that might help you move things forward?

Helman[8]

Helman's 'folk model' is another model that tries to explain why patients behave the way that they do. Helman was a medical anthropologist who had significant insights into cultural factors that influence health and illness. I (MF) often use a form of this model when I am working overseas and it seems to work well for situations where the doctor comes from a different cultural background to the patient and so is like a fish out of water.* Hence, it may be a particularly useful one to bear in mind if you are coming to the UK with a different cultural heritage. It is very patient centred and concentrates on six questions that the patient wants answering within the consultation, which may or may not be explicitly asked.

The questions are:
1. What has happened?
2. Why has it happened?
3. Why to me?
4. Why now?
5. What would happen if nothing were done about it?
6. What should I do about it or whom should I consult for further help?

Another useful thing to think about when considering this model is that the patient may well have already asked these questions of friends and family. So it is worth exploring what the patient has already concluded and what treatments or strategies he or she may have already tried. Sometimes we are the last link in a chain, or even simply an access point to further care, which may or may not be appropriate for the clinical situation. For example, we can think of many patients, such as those from Eastern Europe, who very much view GPs as gatekeepers to other services, such as gynaecologists, when actually we may be better placed to fulfil their needs.

You may also find it helpful to use this model to identify themes that recur across similar consultations. In particular you may like to consider it with patients who come into the consultation feeling that they may have worked out the why but who don't initially tell you the what! For example, patients may come in with the statement, 'I'm sure it's the weather that's flared things up' and many of these patients may well be referring to joint problems, as it is a commonly held belief in the UK that cold weather makes joints more painful. Knowing this can help you to move the consultation on. However, it is clearly important not to make assumptions, as the patient could equally well be referring to an exacerbation of their hay fever or recurrent migraines when thunder is threatened.

Phrase notes
* 'fish out of water' – being in a behavioural state outside of your comfort zone

WHAT NEXT?

This is by no means an exhaustive description of all the consultation models available, as that is not the focus of this book. We have tried to focus on those that feature as part of the MRCGP exam or those that experience has taught us seem to be the most valuable for OMGs. If you would like more information then there are several texts available that look into this area in more detail.

Suggestions for further reading:
- to get a more detailed perspective on each model described here, *see* source texts listed in the References section.

For a broad sweep across more models:
- Moulton L. *The Naked Consultation: a practical guide to primary care consultation skills*. Oxford: Radcliffe Publishing; 2007.
- Mehay R, Beaumont R, Draper J, *et al. Revisiting models of the consultation*. Online chapter within *The Essential GP Training Handbook*. Oxford: Radcliffe Publishing; 2012. Available at: www.essentialgptrainingbook.com/resources/web_chapter_04/04%20consultation%20models.pdf

You may also like to consider ways of constructing the consultation that refer to specific situations. An example of this might be using the SPIKES approach to breaking bad news, which has six distinct steps.[13]
1. S – **Setting** up the interview. This is about ensuring that you have the necessary privacy and time to undertake the consultation. It may also involve allowing the patient to include someone else, such as his or her spouse.
2. P – assessing the patient's **Perception**. This is about finding out what the patient already knows. It involves finding this out directly from the patient, not just relying on information from other clinicians, such as a specialist's letter.
3. I – obtaining the patient's **Invitation**. This is about getting permission from the patient to give him or her more information. Most patients do want to know more but some will not be ready for the news at this point in time. You can sometimes get a sense of this if there appears to be a discrepancy between what the patient tells you, his or her perception, and information from others. It may also relate to the interview not having been set up properly and the patient wanting someone else to be present (or, occasionally, absent).
4. K – giving **Knowledge**. This is about imparting information to the patient. It should include a warning shot rather than launching straight into the bad news. You also need to divide the information into small chunks, allowing time for both silence and emotions. Trying to mirror the patient's use of language can be very effective.
5. E – addressing **Emotions**. You need to be able to recognise the emotions that

the patient displays and identify both their cause and effect. This is about exploring emotions and empathising with the patient.

6. S – **Strategy** and **Summary**. Having a clear plan for the future can really help to reduce the patient's anxiety and fear. This stage involves summarising the discussion so far and what happens next. It may be as simple as setting up the next interview or may be a more complex discussion on the treatment options available and needs to be tailored to what a particular patient is ready to hear.

Another example of a particular construct might be the BATHE[14] approach to patients who are psychologically distressed.

Background – seeking to establish the context for the patient's visit:
● *'What is going on in your life?'*

Affect – getting the patient to report on his or her current feelings and mood:
● *'How do you feel about that?'*

Trouble – finding out how the situation is affecting the patient:
● *'What in particular is troubling you about that?'*

Handling – finding out what strategies the patient is already using, or has thought of:
● *'How have you been handling that?'*

Empathy – showing the patient that you are concerned for him or her:
● *'That must be very difficult for you'*

These are just two examples of constructs that you can use for particular situations. Perhaps you can think of other situations that you find challenging? Common examples might be conflict situations with angry patients or ethical dilemmas. If these situations tend to make you panic, like a rabbit in the headlights, then it may be worth you exploring what constructs are available, or even trying to devise your own. This will then give you something to fall back on when faced with such situations, be it in an exam setting or in everyday practice.

The most important thing to remember when considering approaches to the consultation is that, in the same way that patients are all different individuals, so too are we as doctors. There is no easy solution, or one-size-fits-all. The point of having consultation models and constructs is about equipping us with a toolkit of different approaches to use in different situations. The skill comes with knowing what to use when, just as a skilled craftsman knows when it is appropriate to use power tools and when a more delicate approach is required. Developing these skills comes with experience and practice and also with increasing our self-awareness as to what it is about us that influences a particular situation.

REFERENCES

1. Launer J. *Narrative-Based Primary Care: a practical guide*. Radcliffe Medical Press: Oxford; 2002.
2. Kenny D. A consultation navigation tool: an aid for teaching consultation skills. *Educ Prim Care*. 2012; **23**(1): 41–3.
3. Neighbour R. *The Inner Consultation: how to develop an effective and intuitive consulting style*. 2nd ed. LibraPharm Limited: Newbury; 2004.
4. Pendelton P, Schofield T, Tate P, *et al. The Consultation: an approach to learning and teaching*. Oxford University Press: Oxford; 1984.
5. Stott NC, Davis RH. The exceptional potential into each primary care consultation. *J R Coll Gen Pract*. 1979; **29**(201): 201–5.
6. Tuckett D, Boulton M, Olson C, *et al. Meetings between Experts: an approach to sharing ideas in medical consultations*. London: Routledge; 1985.
7. Byrne PS, Long BEL. *Doctors Talking to Patients*. London: HMSO; 1976.
8. Helman CG. Disease versus illness in general practice. *J R Coll Gen Pract*. 1981; **31**(230): 548–52.
9. Berne E. *Games People Play: the psychology of human relationships*. London: The Penguin Group;1964.
10. Balint M. *The Doctor, his patient and the illness*. Edinburgh: Churchill Livingstone;1957.
11. Levenstein JH, McCracken EC, McWhinney IR, *et al.* The patient-centred clinical method: 1. A model for doctor-patient interaction in family medicine. *Fam Pract*. 1986; **3**(1): 24–30.
12. Silverman J, Kurtz SM, Draper J. *Skills for Communicating with Patients*. Oxford: Radcliffe Medical Press;1996.
13. Baile WF, Buckman R, Lenzi R, *et al.* SPIKES—a six-step protocol for delivering bad news: application to the patient with cancer. *Oncologist*. 2000; **5**(4): 302–11.
14. McCulloch J, Ramesar S, Peterson H. Psychotherapy in primary care: the BATHE technique. *Am Fam Physician*. 1998; **57**(9): 2131–4.

CHAPTER 4

Language, culture and communication: enhancing the patient–doctor dialogue

Anneliese Guerin-LeTendre

INTRODUCTION

In this chapter we'll be looking at what makes us good communicators. We will question a number of platitudes about communication, especially the one that says: 'Communication is just about using the language correctly'. Many doctors who come from abroad to train as GPs in the UK find that the professional role, and the CSA examination, present cultural and linguistic challenges that they had not anticipated. The intention in including this chapter is to prepare you for these challenges.

We'll think about what we mean by 'good' or 'effective 'communication, how interpersonal communication works, and why it can sometimes break down in the consultation room. We'll be taking some examples from your professional experience – and you will pick up ideas and strategies, which you can apply immediately in your role as a GP. You will find more ideas and suggestions for further reading at the end of the chapter.

As in the other chapters in this book, there will be regular 'Action Points', which will provide opportunities for you to reflect on your current practice and ways in which you can continue to enhance your skills. Since it is impossible in this context to separate language and culture, there will also be occasional 'Culture Notes' to support your observations and learning.

We will be working on the assumption that you are working with English speakers. We know of course that one of the defining features of the UK is its cultural diversity – and you are a part of it. So this entire chapter is really about intercultural communication. Nevertheless, your interaction with your patients and colleagues will be shaped by the cultural tendencies or preferences – norms of behaviour, assumptions and values – that are typical of the UK. This necessarily means that we will need to generalise a little; as in any culture, there are those who conform exactly to the typical profile, others less so, and still others not at all!

Of course good medical practice is based on treating all patients equally, regardless of cultural background – religious, ethnic, social … Understanding this diversity is essential for effective communication and therefore a challenge for all doctors working in the UK. However, coming from abroad, you may find yourself in an even more challenging position because of the differences in education and training you have experienced and the different working practices in your home country.

What is effective communication?

When a doctor establishes a good rapport with his or her patient, shows an ability to listen attentively and give clear explanations, is understood and gets the hoped-for response from his or her patient, then that is considered to be effective interpersonal communication. Therefore, effective communication brings together linguistic skill and emotional connection (usually referred to as emotional intelligence or 'EQ') for a successful doctor–patient relationship.

Interpersonal communication is often described as a 'soft skill' – which makes it sound like something rather vague – and quite easy compared with the technical 'hard skills', which fields such as engineering and medicine require. The reality, as you have probably already discovered, is that communication is the most demanding of all our skills – requiring intellectual, emotional and even physical mindfulness!

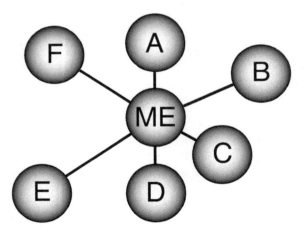

FIGURE 4.1 As the speaker, we feel at the centre of what's going on

When we are talking with others we often tend to think of ourselves at the centre of what is happening. People move around us, coming into focus and then receding from view, but basically we're at the heart of it all, and in control! Naturally, in large organisations such as hospitals, daily routine, work life and communication feels very different to the atmosphere in smaller work communities such as general practice, where there are generally fewer points of interaction, and fewer people to interact with at any one time. Some doctors find the atmosphere of general practice more comfortable, while others find working in a busy hospital department more exhilarating. Whatever our work context, we still tend to have the impression that our communication with others should work something like the diagram in Figure 4.2.

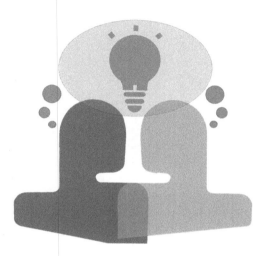

FIGURE 4.2 Our intuitive feeling about how communication works

For example, you, the doctor, formulate an idea and convey that idea – diagnosis, recommendation, range of health options, and so forth – in a language spoken by both you and the patient. The patient then understands and responds appropriately. The reality we all know and experience daily is that communication is often more complex than this! One of the earliest and simplest models of communication allows us to see what's happening more clearly (*see* Figure 4.3).

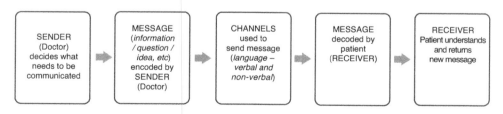

FIGURE 4.3 The 'transmission model' of communication (adapted from Shannon and Weaver, 1949; *see* p. 72)

The transmission model* helps us to see how social interactions can be broken down into component parts and it is then that we begin to see the complexity of communication: how accurately can the messages be transmitted; how precisely can the meaning be conveyed; how effectively does the received meaning affect behaviour? We will return to this question of how we make meaning from what we say and what we hear, and how that interpretation can determine our responses.

However, this model fails to tell us about the quality, or the effectiveness, of the way we communicate! For example, the model is built on the assumption that we always communicate from our own 'bubble' directly to another person's 'bubble'; that the listener is in the same context; that our 'message' is consistently clear; that our listener will immediately know exactly what we mean to say. However, the reality is that this is often not the case.

So how do we bridge the gap in understanding between what people say and what they mean? And how do we know when we're getting it right? Of course, we can look for indicators that will confirm that we have succeeded – a feeling of rapport and shared understanding during a consultation, a feeling of trust and mutual respect with the patient. We'll know we have succeeded if we feel comfortable and confident in the relationship, and we might even anticipate that, as a result of this successful communication, there will be at least the potential for a continuing professional relationship. Above all we'll know our communication has been successful if we have managed to achieve our 'goal' or objective for the interaction: getting a response to a letter of referral, managing a challenging conversation, agreeing a shared management plan with a patient.

Messages are often messed up in the encoding and decoding processes. We sometimes call these decoding errors 'noise'. In a consultation this 'noise' can come from the GP's use of medical jargon, an inappropriate level of formality, from competing (unspoken) messages, from the listener's mistakes in decoding the language (for example, interpreting 'rash' to mean skin cancer), preconceived ideas about the subject being discussed or about the person who is speaking – to mention just a few! In short, we could list many sources of 'noise' or interference in effective communication. As we move through this chapter, you will see more examples.

Even when we are speaking the same language there's often a difference between what we say and what we mean – speaking the same language isn't any guarantee of 'good' communication. Our interactions are sometimes quite straightforward and obvious – the kind of transactional encounter we

---

* This theory, proposed by mathematicians Shannon and Weaver (Shannon C and Weaver W. *The Mathematical Theory of Communication*. Urbana: University of Illinois Press; 1949) was originally intended for use by engineers, in the context of information transmission over telephone lines. Although the theory was originally intended for dealing with information that was void of meaning, the transmission model is still one of the most popular points of reference for interpersonal communication models used today.

have regularly, such as buying a newspaper or a train ticket. Much more often, the conversation moves in unexpected directions, so those participating have to pay attention to the moves of others and be flexible in how they respond. Misunderstandings on many different levels can happen even in small teams, among friends, within families and between partners – people we know, and who know us well!

It's a wonder we manage to communicate at all isn't it? But of course we are social animals and we do communicate, and often, and often brilliantly! We just need to check that we are communicating what we *think* we are communicating (that is, check out the validity of our communication) and develop an awareness of how we can sometimes sabotage even our best intentions.

ACTION POINT 1

- Which of the possible sources of 'noise' mentioned here might interfere with clear communication between you and your patient? Can you think of any other examples?
- What can you do to manage – or avoid – this kind of interference?
- Which of these sources of noise have *in fact* interfered with one of your consultations? Try to remember a specific example connected to a few of these types of noise. On reflection, at what stage along the dialogue did the 'noise' occur? What did you do to rectify the situation?

The interaction of culture and communication

So, communication is complex; we are constantly sending and receiving messages – simultaneously 'translating' and reacting to them, and feeding the responses back into the dialogue. Furthermore, all this is happening within a culture or overlapping cultures – our own individual cultural make-up – composed of the mix of education, ethnic group, religion, social background, and so forth – and the national, organisational, professional cultures within which we live and communicate.

CULTURE NOTE

Each of these cultures (including the culture of the medical profession) has its own strong values, accepted norms of behaviour, clear assumptions about 'how things are' and confident perspectives on the world. None of these cultures is fixed or static; on the contrary, the cultures we move about in are dynamic, 'happening' phenomena, created by the people who inhabit them – you, me, him, her, them and us!

As soon as we walk into a group, a team or an organisation, the culture of that group is subtly changed by our presence. This is what creates the richness of our interactions and the wonderful diversity of all organisations great and small; each person contributes his/her individual qualities, values, experience and perspectives. Also, because we are social animals and born to interact (as

Daniel Goleman says, 'We are hard-wired to connect'[1]), we usually want to make connections with each other, even if we sometimes sabotage our own best efforts!

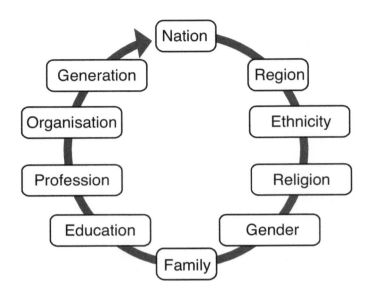

FIGURE 4.4 Our individual culture is made up of many influences

Why effective interpersonal communication matters in the consulting room

It's not quite enough to be a technical medical expert. Research has shown that doctors with 'a good bedside manner' are more effective in terms of patient well-being.[2] The doctor contributes to the physical and mental well-being of his or her patients by engaging patients in precise and clear conversations about healthy lifestyles and behaviours, and by persuading them of the value following a certain treatment or reducing risky behaviours. Of course, clinical skills are the heart of the matter, but irrespective of the medical advances in stem cell research, cellular 'leapfrogging', robot surgery or healthcare 'avatars', the communication skills of healthcare professionals remain crucially important.

ACTION POINT 2

- Which of the skills for effective interpersonal communication do you already bring to your work as a doctor?
- Which skills would you like to develop further?

THOUGHTS ON ... INITIATING THE CONSULTATION
The first encounter

As we said at the beginning of this chapter, all communication takes place within a cultural context. During a medical consultation, the culture of both the doctor and the patient determine how the two parties interact. Even before the consultation begins, your patient will probably have the opportunity to observe you and your relationships with colleagues and other patients. He or she will hear what you say and read your non-verbal communication. This will shape the patient's perception of you and therefore the way in which the relationship develops. When perceptions and expectations are created, the human brain starts using those perceptions and expectations to resolve any knowledge gaps or ambiguity in our interactions with other people: 'This is a funny and effective doctor/an arrogant and condescending doctor/an indifferent doctor/a doctor who cares about people' ... 'I know because of how I see him behave with the receptionists/other patients/the practice nurse'.

CULTURE
NOTE

Non-verbal communication

If we think about it, much of the communication context of the consultation is significantly influenced by the doctor and by the members of the general practice where he or she works – and much of this context is communicated non-verbally. The location, interior design, the furniture (even the magazines in the waiting room!) and the layout of the consulting room are in some way a reflection of the doctor and the team. Those objects we choose to have around us act as symbols – for example, of success, status and identity. Peter Tate[3] suggests how a GP surgery – strange-looking equipment, impressive certificates on the wall, a computer with illegible displays, large desk, big chair, and attached (subservient) staff – might seem intimidating from a patient's point of view. How will you manage the patient's interpretation of these non-verbal cues?

Then there are those very first seconds of the consultation. In this culture, eye contact is considered an indicator of trust and honesty and essential for rapport building. Throughout the consultation, eye contact and the occasional nod will encourage your patient to continue talking. That doesn't mean to say that you will never break eye contact, but if you notice that your patient seems to be avoiding eye contact it might be an indication of discomfort or anxiety. What do you learn from the first few seconds of meeting your patient? I encourage you to pick up as many clues as you can right from the very start of the consultation.

Watch your own body language too. Does it say, 'My focus is on you; you are my only concern for the whole period of this consultation'? This attention will be conveyed partly by eye contact, facial expression and tone of voice, and partly by the way you sit in relation to your patient. Doctors who face their patients, lean forward, sit closer and keep their arms and legs in an open position are perceived as having a high rapport. The 'space bubble', or social distance we adopt in different settings, reflects attraction, comfort or discomfort, status, or the intensity of the exchange. Being too distant is perceived as being cold and unsympathetic; being too close is commonly viewed as intrusive of personal space. Most people in the UK feel comfortable within a relatively large distance – around 1.2 meters of 'space bubble' is considered acceptable between strangers (rather like sitting next to someone with room for another person between you!). This compares with 0.5 meters for family and friends,[4] although of course when you are carrying out physical examinations you will be entering this 'space bubble'.

Sitting at right angles at the corner of your desk and facing your patient, rather than opposite each other across a table, encourages rapport building and makes reading non-verbal signals easier. This will also mean that your patient can see your computer screen if you want to share information – or simply act as an indicator of openness and trust. How will you take notes while trying to focus on the non-verbal communication signals of your patient? Separating listening and note-taking with verbal signalling ('Thank you, I'll just make a quick note of what you've told me so far'), may be the answer for you.

All this sounds outrageously complicated. Don't panic, but just remember that your interpersonal skills as a doctor are considerably enhanced by your awareness of what is being conveyed – by you as well as your patient – through non-verbal communication.

A patient-centred approach

CULTURE
NOTE

Here let's pause to think about the cultural impact on the role of the doctor. You may have come from a culture where the status and role of the doctor is very different to that of the doctor in the UK. As a result of a combination of cultural/social and scientific/clinical factors, the public perception of the status of the doctor has changed. In your culture patients may expect their doctor to provide solutions and tell them what to do rather than discuss options or agree a negotiated plan. For this reason you may well be puzzled by the 'patient-centred' or 'partnership' model of medical practice you are expected to adopt as a GP in the UK. Moreover, if in your home culture the individual has to pay for healthcare, the definition of a 'good' doctor may be one who can diagnose the problem quickly and 'tell' the patient the 'answer' to their health problem, without recourse to further (and probably expensive) treatments, assessments and follow-up appointments.

You may even find this 'egalitarian' cultural preference of the UK stressful; its emphasis on shared decision-making and reaching concordance with the patient might leave you feeling that you're not really doing your job 'properly' according to the way you were trained. Your communication style may well need to 'flex' too. Some patients will arrive in your consultation room informed by ideas gleaned from the internet or other media and will feel confident in challenging your suggestions and advice. In such cases you may have to draw on your negotiation skills more than you have previously in order to persuade and convince your patient of what is in his or her best interests for his or her individual health and well-being. Since respect for professional roles and status is not automatic, your patients won't expect you to use 'distant' and formal language either. Later on I will be making some suggestions that will help you to make your language more informal, but professional, and allow you to still feel like you are 'being yourself'.

Before we leave this topic, it's worth remembering also that not all of your patients will want – or feel able to – share in decision-making in the way described here. Explore the expectations of each individual patient, support them by giving explanations and suggestions, encourage them to take responsibility for their own healthcare – and be prepared to adapt to individual personalities, needs and preferences.

Establishing rapport

In those first few seconds as you greet your patient and give them time to settle down you are setting the tone for good communication (indeed, the first few moments of any interaction can be defining moments for the relationship!). The consultation starts well when your initial greeting, your non-verbal communication and your opening questions come across as confident, warm and not too formal. As you invite your patient into your consultation room you will probably be making 'small talk' – what we call 'phatic communication' – using language to establish a mood of sociability rather than to communicate information. Comments such as 'What a lovely day' or 'At least all this rain is good for the garden', or (if this is a patient you've seen relatively recently) 'How have you been keeping?' are preludes to the real opening question that gets the consultation underway: 'So what brings you here to see me today?'

We've talked a lot about non-verbal communication already, and your ability to read and respond to non-verbal cues is one of the most important skills you can have in your interpersonal communications 'toolkit'. So perhaps now is a good time to reflect on your own non-verbal communication style and how you use it to build rapport.

Timing: get rid of the guilt

Of necessity the consultation will be time-framed by the doctor and the practice – although the needs of individual patients may mean that this time frame has to be extended. You know that on average you will have about 10 minutes to give to each patient. If you come from a culture where there are no such time constraints, this may seem daunting – even impossible to achieve. Interestingly, evidence suggests that there is virtually no correlation between the time spent in a consultation and patient satisfaction or doctor effectiveness.[5] Nevertheless, you may feel nervous about mentioning the limited time available in case the

ACTION POINT 3

- How would you describe your own non-verbal communication?
- What does your body language say about you?
- Try this quiz – perhaps keep a log over a few days, or ask for feedback from friends and colleagues.

Non-verbal communication signals	Always	Sometimes	Never	Remarks
I think that a firm handshake shows strength of character and a positive personality				
I feel comfortable using direct eye contact				
I smile to show I am happy and relaxed, or that I agree				
I think it's important to think about the impression my general appearance gives of me as a doctor				
I generally nod my head slowly from time to time when I am listening carefully				
I make a point of starting and finishing consultations on time				
When speaking I use hand gestures to reinforce my message				
When sitting talking with a patient or colleague I usually sit legs uncrossed and pointed toward the other person				
I feel comfortable with occasional silences during a conversation				

CULTURE NOTE

- From what you have observed, which of these non-verbal signals are considered positive indicators in UK culture? Would these indicators be the same in your own culture?
- You might find it interesting to discuss your observations with colleagues, your trainer and your ES.

patient is irritated or less likely to cooperate fully in the consultation dialogue. In reality, this time focus can be used positively to encourage both doctor and patient to make full use of time available.

Managing your time effectively will ensure that your patient does not feel 'rushed or crushed'. Some cultures view time as infinitely plentiful and flexible, so notions of time (being 'on time, late, early, punctual,' etc.) are subservient to other factors such as commitments involving people and relationships or the weather. In the cultural context of the UK – one of those cultures where time is viewed as a scarce commodity to be used wisely – being punctual, respecting schedules and pre-arranged appointments, is often interpreted as an indication of fairness, courtesy and respect (even if not everyone follows these 'rules'). So you can feel comfortable about trying to keep to the time limit set – negotiating priorities if necessary.

CULTURE NOTE

'Signposting' the different stages of the consultation as you go will help both you and your patient to be aware of the time you both have. When you are both clear about the time available, you and the patient can feel more relaxed and focus on the matter in hand. Good time management will also help you manage your energy. You may even come to the conclusion that working within a time constraint can actually be positive in helping to focus the mind – both yours and that of your patient. Lengthy consultations may not mean that the patient is better able to explain his or her problem – or more likely to remember all the information he or she has been given.

Some patients will arrive with multiple issues to discuss, hoping to make the most of the opportunity of seeing you ('while I'm here …'). In such cases 'signposting' and 'chunking' are useful. First, you will need to agree an agenda, by helping the patient to prioritise.

It sounds like there are a number of things you would like to talk about today. Perhaps you can tell me which are at the top of your list – that way we can deal with the most important things in the time we have today.

OK, so what if we find out first whether one of your medicines is causing your upset stomach? Then we can deal with the eczema on your legs. Is that OK?

Let's deal with … now, and then we'll look at … next.

Bear in mind also that the patient's priority may not be the most pressing priority from a doctor's point of view; you will need to make your own clinical assessment about which of the patient's priorities takes medical precedence.

THOUGHTS ON … INFORMATION GATHERING
Language choice for patient-centred consultations

In any situation where there is potential inequality between people, the language we choose can either reinforce that distance, or bridge the gap. For example, using medical jargon that the patient is unlikely to understand, or downloading huge amounts of information without checking whether the patient wants or needs it, might reinforce your status as 'expert' but will be unlikely to create a feeling of rapport – indeed, it might well leave the patient feeling ignored, frustrated or even angry. Here are some suggestions for creating rapport, gaining the trust of your patient, and so communicating effectively:

- notice the kind of words/language used by the patient and …
- align your language with theirs
- employ diagrams, drawings, visuals, write down key words if necessary
- use plain language as much as possible.

Naturally, if the patient wants or needs to know the medical term, use it and then explain it.

The trick for building rapport is often listening carefully and mirroring some part of what you hear. In this example the doctor is mirroring the patients' communication style:

Patient: It's quite a sharp pain – yesterday I actually *came over* all dizzy when I was at the shops.
Doctor: And when did this pain first *come on*?

'Phrasal verbs' such as those highlighted in the patient–doctor dialogue here can prove useful in consultations; they are often used to create a feeling of informality and friendliness.

As you can see opposite, individual phrasal verbs can have a range of meanings. Let's take the example of phrasal verbs with 'up', which has the connotation of 'high-intensity' change. For example, 'to heal' is to heal normally; 'to heal up' is to heal more quickly; 'to swell' is to grow larger at a pace that is not particularly shocking; 'to swell up' is a much more intense sort of swelling.

Think about how the following verbs have been intensified by the use of 'up':

build up, clear up, flare up, heal up, swell up, take up, tone up.

WHAT ARE 'PHRASAL VERBS'?

Phrasal verbs are made up of a verb + a particle and/or a preposition, or a verb + particle + preposition. For example:

Verb + *preposition*
- Who is <u>looking</u> *after* the children at the moment?
- I've got <u>to fight</u> *off* this cold – I can't afford the time off work!
- I'll give you something to help <u>bring</u> your temperature *down*.
- Don't worry, you'll soon <u>get</u> *over* it.
- She <u>takes</u> *after* her mother.
- My last doctor <u>put</u> me *on* antibiotics.
- The rash on your arm seems to have <u>cleared</u> *up* nicely.
- I'm sorry doctor, can you explain that again – I just can't <u>take</u> anything *in* at the moment.
- I've <u>blacked</u> *out* three times in the last few weeks.
- She refused to eat her dinner; she says she can't <u>keep</u> anything *down*.

Verb + *particle* + *preposition*
- I've got a temperature, a headache, a sore throat … I think <u>I'm coming</u> *down with* the flu.
- It's a bit uncomfortable but I can <u>put</u> *up with* that for a few days.
- My mother's going into respite care for a few days – to be honest <u>I'm looking forward to</u> a rest.
- I'm worried that my <u>son is hanging</u> *out with* the kind of people who take drugs.

The particularity of phrasal verbs is that their meaning cannot be understood by looking at the meaning of their component parts in isolation. So for example if you 'hang out' with friends, you are actually 'spending time' with them, rather than actually hanging from anything! The meaning of the two or more words together is often drastically different from what you might guess it to be based upon the meanings of the individual parts in isolation.

Phrasal verbs can also be changed into nouns (verb + particle before or after the verbs, e.g. Standby:
- I'll *stand by* in case you need me. (verb)
- We are keeping the old equipment on *standby*, in case of emergency. (noun)
  Breakdown:
- She was obviously very upset – in fact she *broke down* in tears. (verb)
- He's suffering from enormous stress at work – I'm worried he might be heading for a nervous *breakdown*. (noun)

You'll notice the difference because of the changes in stress patterns as verbs change to nouns.

Here are a couple more examples to show how the doctor uses phrasal verbs to create a feeling of rapport.

Doctor: How's that knee *coming along*?
Patient: Well, the consultant said I'd *come through* the operation quite well but I don't feel I've *got over* it yet.
Doctor: Well, it'll take a while to *settle down*, but the exercises will help.

Patient: I think I'm *coming down* with something – I keep *throwing up* and I've *come out* in red spots.
Doctor: Hmm, let's *have a look at* those spots … have you thought about what this might be?

ACTION POINT 4

Take your smartphone (or, if you prefer, a notebook or Post-it block – something you can keep handy). List the seven most useful phrasal verbs you already use or hear used during consultations – you could start with the list given earlier – and make a point of introducing them as appropriate.

If, as you go through your day, you read or hear examples that could be especially useful in your consultation, jot down these expressions and use them as soon as there is an opportunity.

Correct use of these little verbs will distinguish you as a confident English speaker, add to your credibility and help build rapport.

Asking questions

In view of the limited time available in the consultation, you may want to 'play safe' by having a ready-made list of questions in your mind. Of course your questioning has to be purposeful, and it's tempting to think that being able to rattle off a quick-fire succession of questions will elicit the information you need as 'efficiently' as possible.

However, do bear in mind the risks involved in this approach:

- possible break-down in rapport – your patient will certainly notice he or she is being rushed
- less focus on listening – you risk repeating questions that the patient has already answered
- overlooking vital patient cues – relying too heavily on a formulaic approach to asking questions may lead you to focus on diagnosis too early.

So make every question count. For example, when using the ICE model (Ideas, Concerns and Expectations), consider the value of pursuing the patient for his or her opinion about a possible diagnosis, treatment or prognosis; if the patient really doesn't seem to know or isn't able or willing to give an answer, just move on.

Of course, everybody has some thoughts on health, but asking direct questions may not always be the best way to elicit a 'real' answer. Some alternative suggestions are outlined here.

Vary questioning techniques: combine open and closed questions

Encourage the patient to talk	'People usually have some sort of idea about their illness. What have you been thinking?'	'What were you hoping to get out of our meeting today?'
Explain why you need to know	'I was wondering whether this might be because …'	'Have you noticed …? I was thinking it might be…'
Use softeners to show sensitivity (to the British ear)	'I was wondering …' 'It's interesting that …' 'Understandably …'	'Would you mind if …' 'Now what if you could …' 'I'm curious about …'
Share 'anecdotes' – real or invented – to encourage your patient to talk	'I had a patient once a bit like you – he had to go through this same operation too – and I wondered how you were feeling about it?'	'Now I don't know if you're the kind of person who, like my friend Kathleen, could stop smoking on a £10 bet!'
Use open questions to allow the patient to give a more complete answer	'Tell me about these headaches you've been having.'	'What makes them better or worse?'
… but note that open questions sometimes require time management	'I think we have enough information to go on for the time being. Let's have a listen to your heart.'	'Great – I think I get the picture: you are saying that … So let's see what we can do about this.'
Choose closed questions when you want short answers, in order to obtain and classify more precise information and/or establish a pattern	**Doctor**: How long do your headaches last? **Patient**: An hour.	**Doctor**: Do you ever wake up with a headache in the morning? **Patient**: Yes. **Doctor**: How often does that happen? **Patient**: Most mornings.
Use more closed questions than open questions toward the end of the information gathering and let your patient know that you are about to do so	'Would it be OK if I asked you some specific questions now?'	'I just need to ask you a few more details about …'

Open questioning techniques place the patient at the centre of the consultation, as the expert of his or her own health problem and the main source of information (including the expression of emotions and feelings). Open questions can also drastically reduce the number of questions you need to ask; they may even elicit information that you would not otherwise have found out. Generally speaking, the more closed questions and leading questions there are, the more the consultation will be 'doctor centred'.

Pros and cons of asking 'leading' questions

Leading questions focus on finding out a specific point or detail	'Does the pain always come on after exercise?'	Compare with: 'When does the pain usually come on?' or 'Tell me more about this pain'
Leading questions can be counterproductive	'So you're worried about your operation coming up?'	Compare with: 'How are you feeling about the operation?' where the patient is given the freedom to express his or her feelings
Sometimes leading questions don't sound like questions at all but, rather, they are statements used to express empathy	'It must be difficult coping with your mother-in-law and the children' 'I bet you're feeling exhausted' 'That must have been disappointing for you' 'You must be in a lot of pain'	These expressions of empathy show that you are putting yourself in their shoes; they often begin with 'it must' or 'you must' and sometimes 'I bet'
… and using statements as questions also gives the patient an opportunity to respond – especially when emotions are difficult to express or the subject is sensitive Here pausing after the statement is essential	'I was wondering whether … (you have ever thought about going to a counsellor) + pause Some people find … (that going to a support group is helpful) + pause It's difficult to … (change the habits of a lifetime) + pause I can see this is very difficult for you … (+ pause)	Allow the patient time to respond to the remark Acknowledge the patient's feelings, offer support and give the patient time to regain his or her composure

As you know, the quality of your questions will determine the quality of the whole consultation but keep comparing what you are hearing with the non-verbal communication you are observing.

Doctor: Is there anything particular worrying you?
Patient: Er … no, I don't think so [*breaking eye contact*].

What kind of body language might you expect with 'I'm fine' or 'Work's going well'?

Don't forget that the implicit rules governing conversation stipulate that questions, if not answered, then need to at least be responded to in some way – even if the response is merely 'masquerading' as an answer. Therefore, you may need to ask further probing questions to gain the level of detail you need.

Allow time for your patient to ask questions too – and notice how he or she asks the question.

Asking multiple questions can cause confusion

Multiple questions usually consist of an open question used to provide context, followed by at least one or sometimes two closed questions to elicit the specific information required.	'So can you describe this pain for me? When did it come on? Do you have this pain now? 'How have you been feeling since your operation? Are you eating? Do you have a good appetite?'	There is nothing inherently wrong in this kind of questioning in some contexts, but in a consultation, multiple questions risk confusing your patient. Which question should the patient answer first? Can the patient remember all the questions and line up his or her answers accordingly? You may find that the patient simply answers the final question, in which case you will only have some of the information you were looking for. If you have a number of questions in mind, ask them one at a time, allowing the patient time to answer.

Choosing question styles

To summarise, during the course of the consultation you will gradually move from open questioning techniques to more directive questions and statements in order to guide the patient to give more information about specific details. However, it is important not to be too quick to jump ahead to closed questions to test your own (possibly premature) hypothesis. Open questions will enable you to gather detailed background information about past medical history, family history, personal and social background, medication and allergy history. As the consultation progresses you will be asking increasingly directed questions in order to focus on specific details, finally finishing with closed questions before moving on to the physical examination, the diagnosis and the shared plan. Thinking about different ways of eliciting information from your patients will keep your consultations fresh, encourage good rapport and help you to maintain a patient-centred approach.

ACTION POINT 5

- Think about your questioning techniques. Draw up a checklist of possible questioning techniques for eliciting ideas, concerns, expectations and feelings; use it to review your consultations over a period of a week, or a given number of consultations (don't forget you can use 'softeners' too).
- Next, decide to try out some different approaches over the period of a week. What do you observe?
- Discuss your observations with your supervisor, trainer and colleagues. What do you want, or need, to do next?

Picking up on patient cues

CULTURE
NOTE

As mentioned earlier, in most cases the British tend to favour communication that is direct, explicit and concise, although there are regional variations – Northerners have a reputation for directness, Southerners for being more indirect. However, when it comes to being polite, many British people become very indirect in their communication. In these situations both speaker and listener share the 'secret' of what is going on and are complicit in the way they interact. This politeness is not just about being courteous, but often to do with saving face (yes, just like the Japanese!), avoiding difficult conversations about sensitive issues, not imposing on other people or invading their privacy. (This notion of politeness even extends to not invading personal space; that's why you'll sometimes hear British people apologising for colliding with someone in the street, even though it was the other person who wasn't looking where he was going! You might want to read more about this in Kate Fox's interesting and entertaining book *Watching the English.*[6])

British people consider that being polite and considerate toward one another is one of the defining characteristics of the British.[*] Not surprisingly, these politeness formulae – understatement, self-deprecation, use of humour – support and reinforce a range of British values:

- *modesty* – often conveyed by self-deprecation ('boasting about personal achievements or successes is a sign of arrogance')
- *stoicism in the face of difficulties* – often conveyed by humour ('keep calm and carry on')
- *emotional restraint* – as in the expression 'keep a stiff upper lip' – often conveyed by understatement ('since we found out about my mum's cancer we're finding it *quite* difficult to keep going …')

However, as with all cultural norms of behaviour, not everyone you meet will be polite! What does all this mean in the context of your consultations? Listen out for patients using understatement as a way of making light of their own pain, anxiety, unhappiness, and so forth, in order not to discomfort the listener or impose on the listener's feelings in any way.

Doctor: I'm so sorry to hear that your father passed away.
Patient: Thank you. It's been *a bit* of a struggle for all of us.

---

[*] This is one of the findings from the British Social Attitudes survey from 2005. If you are curious to find out more about the British and how they live, this is a fascinating source. Every year the British Social Attitudes survey asks over 3000 people what it's like to live in Britain and what they think about how Britain is run. Just log on to the survey website (www.bsa-30.natcen.ac.uk).

Certain words and phrases are used to lessen the impact of what is being said (this is called 'hedging'):

insignificant problem / *somewhat* disappointed / *a bit* concerned / *slightly* worrying / *kind of* complicated / *minor* twinges / *one or two* problems …

ACTION POINT 6

Here are some examples of patients using understatement. What do they really mean? Listen out for patients and colleagues using these words to downplay their real feelings:

She's been *pretty* off-colour for the last week now.
I felt *slightly* troubled when I first got the results.
I'm feeling *fairly* exhausted at the moment.
I'm *quite* worried about how my husband might react.
I've been feeling *a bit* rough lately.
I've been feeling *rather* done-in for the last week or so.

Substituting the word 'very' will often give you the real intended meaning.

Looking out for 'micro-messaging'

Small involuntary gestures such as glancing at your watch while someone is speaking, leaning forward during a conversation with a colleague, briefly breaking eye contact, adjusting your position in your chair ('fidgeting'), the pupils of the eyes contracting, an eyebrow lift, corner of the mouth twitch – are examples of what is sometimes referred to as 'micro-messaging'. In an average 10-minute conversation, two people will exchange between 40 and 100 micro-messages.[7] These are less under conscious control than other kinds of non-verbal communication, and therefore will differ more according to cultures. However, as with all non-verbal communication, any kind of mismatch between what we see and what we hear can alert our attention to the real thoughts and feelings of the speaker.

Look at your patient as he or she is talking and develop the habit of 'noticing' any apparent mismatches between the words and the non-verbal signals. Hesitations, changes in tone of voice, loss of eye contact, shifting of position, and 'backing away' movements may be indicators that your patient is 'self-censoring' information – in other words, making conscious decisions about what he or she will, or will not, tell you. Think about what this self-censoring might mean. What might be lying behind this behaviour?

Tapping into your intuition

Research by the psychologist and communication expert Albert Mehrabian[8] suggests that when communicating emotion, we rely on only a tiny proportion of words in order to understand the message (*see* Figure 4.5).

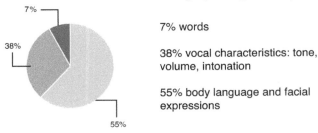

7% words

38% vocal characteristics: tone, volume, intonation

55% body language and facial expressions

FIGURE 4.5 Non-verbal communication (source: Albert Mehrabian, *Non-Verbal Communication*[8])

Anthropological research since the 1950s has demonstrated that certain basic facial expressions – that of happiness, sadness, fear, disgust, surprise and danger – are universally recognisable irrespective of culture, and that the use and recognition of these expressions is genetically inherited rather than socially conditioned or learnt.[9] Taken individually, non-verbal messages can seem ambiguous, but it is important to remember that these codes do not usually function independently or sequentially but, rather, as 'clusters' of behaviour.

- *Crossed arms?* Possibly defensive 'barrier' or the person is feeling cold, or possibly just comfortable sitting that way.
- *Crossed arms and crossed legs?* May be on the defensive, or irritated, but this will need checking out.
- *Crossed legs, crossed arms, frowning, and clenched fists?* Definitely defensive, anticipate anger outburst.

Naturally, as with all interpersonal communications, we also need to interpret meaning according to the individual, the context and the cultural backgrounds of those involved in the dialogue. However, if you see any signs of mismatch between the words and the non-verbal communication, check it out. Open up the dialogue by sharing your observations with your patient:

> I get the feeling ... You seem ... You sound ... You look ... Am I right in thinking that ...?
> I sense that ... I get the impression that ... I notice that ... so can you tell me how you're feeling about ...?

Using 'active listening' techniques

The very word 'listening' (as opposed to 'hearing') suggests active participation on the part of the listener – a conscious effort to connect with the speaker. That positive intention can, however, be sabotaged, or at least undermined, by a lack of awareness of the context of the interaction. The context is not just the location, the setting, the subject and purpose of the consultation, but also the cultural context – background, values, priorities, attitudes, and so forth, of the people involved, which in turn impact on the way in which they interact.

So the use of the expression 'active' listening may seem curious – after all, if we're really listening, it can only be 'active'; however, the label is perhaps useful if it reminds us of the very special effort it takes to really 'listen'. Active listening requires of us that we pay attention in a particularly focused way, and that we be aware of how our own priorities, perceptions, assumptions and judgements can create 'noise' that will interfere with our listening if we let it. As the psychologist Carl Rogers[10] said:

> The greatest barrier to effective communication is the tendency to evaluate what the other person is saying and therefore to misunderstand or to not really 'hear'.

Merely waiting to interrupt with a comment or a question, or lining up a list of possible solutions, or thinking about the next appointment, or the noise outside, or trying to take notes – you get the idea – is not fully paying attention! Listening in the context of a consultation requires looking at the speaker, so that you can pick up on important non-verbal cues and notice not just 'what' your patient is saying but 'how' he or she is saying it. Also notice the order in which the patient is telling you his or her story – does this tell you anything about your patient's priorities?

What the patient says	Echo what the patient says	Paraphrase and summarise what the patient says	Reflect back the possible emotion behind what the patient is saying	Use a question tag
	Pick up key words in the statement and allow the speaker to respond	So what you're saying is/so/if I understand you correctly	Mirror the emotion/ the content sounds like/what I'm hearing is/I get the feeling that	(Don't you/are you/ aren't you/is he/ isn't he/doesn't it/ isn't it/won't you/ haven't you …?)
Example:				
'I don't know how I'm going to cope if my husband gets any worse.'	How you're going to cope? If you're husband gets any worse?	So you're really worried about how you'll manage if your husband's condition continues to get worse	It sounds like you're anxious about what the future holds	It's a very worrying time for you, isn't it? You're feeling up against it right now, aren't you?

Focusing on being fully 'present' when we are listening isn't just about being quiet. All sorts of brain activity is going on as we try to interpret words, tone and body language, distinguish between what is being said and what is being implied, to separate issues that are trivial from those that are significant, to distinguish thoughts and feelings, facts and interpretations. In your consultation you will be using a range of listening techniques to explore what your patient really means. The previous example illustrates how the doctor might use echoing, paraphrasing and summarising, pick up on the emotion or add a question tag to a statement.

Used appropriately, these listening skills can help to build rapport with your patients. What you learn through this kind of attentive listening will enable you to ask relevant questions – which will make it easier for you to identify and respond to your patient's needs more effectively.

Our responses in a conversation also include saying nothing at all; that is, not just being quiet but actually allowing pauses for periods of silence. Think about the reasons for silences within your consultations; perhaps your patient is embarrassed, unsure how to express his or her thoughts and feelings, trying to control emotion, or merely collecting his or her thoughts. Elderly patients and children may take longer to tell their story and you may need to give them some support, express concern or provide gentle encouragement. One way or another a silence will usually indicate that the patient is thinking and feeling something, so allow a little time to elapse before jumping in.

CULTURE NOTE

Knowing when to be silent – in order to give your patient 'space' to talk – can sometimes be difficult, especially when there are time constraints. In 'Anglo-Saxon' cultures like the UK, silence is often interpreted negatively as a breakdown in communication or a sign of disapproval or rejection of an idea. Consequently, we tend not to be very good at allowing a period of silence to elapse and often have an irrepressible urge to fill the gap. Consequently, our interactions tend to resemble a tennis match rather than a game of bowls – you will notice people rushing to cover up breaks in conversation, even in situations like consultations where silences might be appropriate.

Perhaps your own culture feels more comfortable with a slower pace of interaction, with frequent, even long, pauses. If so, you might want to nurture this cultural preference as one of the natural talents you bring to your work. If, like the British, jumping in to fill the gap is your cultural default mode too, try to resist the temptation! A study by Beckman and Frankel[11] found that on average, doctors interrupted after a mean time of 18 seconds – and that 94% of all interruptions resulted in the doctor taking over the consultation altogether. They also found that when the patient was allowed to complete his or her opening statement there was a significant reduction in late-arising problems, making the overall consultation more effective.

Establishing clarity

Look out for generalisations, deletions and distortions.[12] This kind of vague language, if unexplored, can frequently lead to misunderstandings; it encourages the speaker to make sweeping statements, and leaves the listener to make sense of what has been said in any way he or she can or that suits him or her.

Generalisations – using words like all, never, every, none, always, everyone:
- 'I always get a cold in winter.' (Every winter? The same cold throughout?)
- 'Your receptionists are rude.' (Which receptionist said what to you, when and in what circumstances?)

Deletions – some details essential to a complete understanding have been left out:
- 'You can do that easily.' (Possibly, but how exactly?)
- 'Something will have to be done.' (What will have to be done? Who should do it?)

Distortions – turning actual behaviour and events into abstract concepts:
- 'I need help.' (What do you mean by 'help'? In practical terms, what would you have to do in order to feel helped?)

Take the opportunity to explore these and other verbal clues.
- *'It's my back again.'* ('Again'? When was the last time? How long ago? Treatment at that time? Effective or not? Further investigations required?)
- *'My husband thought I ought to come and see you about these headaches I've been having.'* ('Ought'? Her husband encouraged her to come – was there a reason for her reluctance to come? 'These headaches' – so lots of headaches? – How many? How often? 'I've been having' – present perfect progressive verb indicating recent and continuing situation* – since when?)
- (While giving history of physical complaints) *'I've been getting very upset recently.'* ('Upset'? What does that really mean – anxious, tearful, frustrated? 'Recently' – since when?)
- *'I'm giving up smoking.'* ('I am giving up' – present continuous verb. So has he given up yet? No. Explore possible reasons holding him back, when does he intend to start? What support might he need?)

Idiomatic expressions and colloquialisms

It's very likely that when you take up your first post you'll come across idiomatic expressions and colloquialisms that you haven't met before. Indeed, there are so many regional variations – even in the relatively small geographical area of the UK – that even people born in Britain don't know and understand them all! Don't hesitate to pick up on expressions and words you are not familiar with – checking meanings of idiomatic expressions and colloquialisms will not

CULTURE
NOTE

---

* If you ever want to check up on verb tenses and their uses in English, try this handy website: <u>www.englishtenses.com/</u>

undermine your credibility with your patient, but pretending you understand when you don't is a risky strategy! (You will find some examples of commonly used idioms and colloquialisms in Appendix 2, although this is not intended to be, nor could it ever be, an exhaustive list.) Of course the context of the conversation will give you a clue, as well as the non-verbal communication signals, but try echoing them back so that you can be sure of what the patient means.

Patient: I'm feeling generally below par at the moment.
Doctor: Below par?
Patient: Yes, er I just don't feel well, I ...

Patient: I'm all at sixes and sevens about this operation.
Doctor: Sixes and sevens?
Patient: That's right – basically I just don't know what to think, I'm totally confused ...

Patient: Well, Doctor, you see I've been having these funny turns ...
Doctor: Funny turns?
Patient: Well, you know, I go all dizzy and faint like and have to sit down for a while.

Patient: My wife had a bit of a hissy fit when I told her I might have to go into hospital.
Doctor: How do you mean, a hissy fit?
Patient: Well, she went into a bit of a panic like ...

(In the examples above, you will also notice that when people are searching for words because they are finding it hard to explain what they mean, they will often use 'gap fillers' such as *like, you know, basically, I mean, well, it's like* as well as sounds such as *er* and *um*.) Another way of checking for meaning is to come back on expressions the patient has used and ask for specific clarification:

Patient: I haven't been feeling too hot recently.
Doctor: When you say you haven't been feeling that hot, what have you noticed?

Patient: My waterworks have really been playing up ...
Doctor: You said your waterworks have been playing up, can you tell me a bit more about that?

Patient: I feel generally het up.
Doctor: Can you describe what you mean by 'het up'?
Patient: Well, I'm not myself ... since my wife passed away [*died*], everything's gone pear-shaped.

Doctor: Hmm … It's been 6 months now since your wife died, hasn't it? This must be a very difficult time for you. You say 'everything's gone pear-shaped' – how have you been managing?

There are a number of expressions to describe being unwell:

off-colour; off; under the weather; poorly; run down; out of sorts; not that brilliant; not that hot; below par, down in the mouth …

Patients may also use colloquialisms when describing their symptoms – particularly if they are talking about sensitive or very personal issues:

'I'm having problems down below …' (usually vulval/vaginal area)
'Will I need to bring in a sample of water?' (urine)
'I have noticed some white stuff …' (discharge).

When using idiomatic expressions yourself, remember that idiomatic language relies heavily on accuracy and (appropriate) context; start collecting examples so that you understand those most likely to be used by your patients, but check out uses and meanings in other contexts before introducing them into your professional communication.

ACTION POINT 7

If you can, take a few seconds at the end of the consultation to jot down new expressions as you come across them.

Take every opportunity to extend your language skills into more informal and colloquial language.

Group the expressions together into contexts as you hear them being used. For example, words and expressions to do with drug culture:

- to give up drugs without any form of treatment (such as methadone) – kick the habit, detox, clean up, dry out, go cold turkey
- language used to describe negative effects of drug taking – bombed, come down, crash, have a bad trip, have the shakes
- language used to describe the positive effects of drug taking – on a high, spaced out, stoned, wasted, wrecked.

Being a good listener takes energy, concentration and determination, doesn't it?! Listening without judging (so easy to say, but often so hard to do) means disengaging from our own 'world view' with our own assumptions, values and priorities. This way we can be free to focus on what the other person is saying. This doesn't mean abandoning our principles and values, but just not allowing them to become the 'noise' that will interfere with our listening. Don't be surprised if you find the kind of listening you are doing as a GP particularly exhausting on some days – watch out for signs of dropping energy levels and reduced concentration while you are listening and make a conscious effort to refocus as necessary.

ACTION POINT 8

- Observe and reflect on your own listening style – including body language, responses and energy levels. What are your listening strengths? What are your own particular 'roadblocks' to listening? What would you like to change?
- Can you think of examples of patients 'self-censoring'? What were the non-verbal clues? Keep a note of similar examples in your portfolio or personal journal.

THOUGHTS ON … THE PHYSICAL EXAMINATION

This is a time when your patient might feel particularly uncomfortable. Remember what we said earlier about the 'space bubble'? If the doctor needs to come into that intimate space, emotions may range from embarrassment, to discomfort, to feelings of extreme vulnerability; some patients may even feel threatened. How we feel about personal space and our willingness to invite people we do not know into that space depends on our mental and physical state at the time, our previous experiences, and our cultural (including religious) background. Remember to signal to your patient that you are moving on to a physical examination, tell the patient what you are going to do, and why. Again you can use 'softeners' – just, simply, possibly, perhaps – to make the request sound less of an imposition on the other person:

Could you just …? Perhaps you could …?

Here, as throughout the consultation, using inclusive and indirect language for instructions and requests can create rapport, put the patient at ease and reduce embarrassment and anxiety.

Remember that touch is a powerful form of non-verbal communication and associated with strong emotions. Every culture has its own rules about bodily contact and different interpretations of the meaning of touch vary between cultures. For the doctor, touch is probably the most important non-verbal behaviour because of its function in diagnosis and treatment; for example, the doctor will feel the size, shape and location of a lump. You will perhaps be able to make a professional judgement about a patient's potential reaction from his or her ethnic background, religion, gender or age, but check with the patient what feels comfortable for him or her – and, when carrying out intimate physical examinations, always offer a chaperone. Remember also that such examinations must be justified in the context of the clinical problem and supported by the GMC guidelines on good medical practice. If a patient is upset it might feel normal to put your arm around them or place your hand on their shoulder; however often you may find that a particular gesture, such as offering a crying patient a box of tissues, conveys a similar level of empathy without the same potential for misunderstanding.

ACTION POINT 9

Here are some examples of language for polite instructions.

Can/could you + infinitive …?	Could you just *stand up for me* now?
	Can you *sit with your legs stretched out in front of you*?
Would you mind + –ing?	Would you mind *bending your right knee now*?
If you can + infinitive …	If you can try to *bend your left knee now*
I want you to/I'd like you to + infinitive … for me	I want you to *take a deep breath* for me
	I'd like you to *tilt your head forward* for me
Just …	Just *roll up your sleeve*
I need you to …	I need you to *lift your leg as high as you can*

- Try giving the same instructions without the polite 'softeners' (just using the words italicised). Do you notice the difference in tone? Now they sound almost like commands or orders!
- Using the suggestions provided here, try using indirect language and polite instructions for the following: bring your knee up to your chest/press down/breathe out/relax/straighten/bend/lift and lower your arm.

THOUGHTS ON … EXPLAINING THE DIAGNOSIS
Avoiding 'med-speak'

Although medical language is a highly efficient way of transmitting precise information in a short time, studies show that jargon confuses and alienates patients, often leading to misunderstandings. We've said that most of the time it's best to avoid medical jargon in your consultations unless a patient specifically wants to know the 'technical' words. You know the sort of jargon you can dispense with immediately:

- erythema = a redness of the skin
- renal = kidney
- neuropathy = disease of the nerves

- TIA = transient ischaemic attack, a mini-stroke – symptoms that warn of a minor or full stroke
- nephrology department = kidney doctor's clinic.

There are thousands more. Using strings of such terms can make life much more difficult for your patient, whose life is deeply affected by what you are not communicating. It's so easy to lapse into med-speak – and, indeed, when you are talking with colleagues, using jargon is an obvious and useful shorthand. However, like any professional jargon, this 'insider' language excludes people who are not in your professional club!

If you need to use the technical term, give the simple term first and then follow up with an explanation:

Your results show that you have the early stages of diabetes. Let me explain …

Of course, from time to time, the technical word will come to you so much more quickly than its deceptively simple synonym. When that happens, there are simple expressions in English to introduce an explanation and check understanding (*see* Action Point 10).

ACTION POINT 10

Here are examples of how to introduce explanations and check that your patient has understood. Which ones do you remember using in a consultation?

Give explanation	*Check understanding*
that means	Does that make sense?
in other words …	Do you see what I mean?
it's like …	OK so far?
for example …	Do you get the general picture?
to put it another way …	Are you with me?

Using med-speak also encourages an over-reliance on nouns (as jargon is often made up of nouns) that can make your communication less concise and therefore harder to follow. One of the conveniences of using noun-based structures is that it reduces the range of verbs you need to use to those verbs you picked up when you first learnt English. Verbs like to do, to have, to be, to make and to get (generally overused by native English speakers too) are pressed into service when it would be quicker and clearer to use a more precise verb for the exact meaning, in that context:

- You **had** a cutaneous erythematous reaction vs. You broke out in a rash
- There **are** multiple systemic implications of nephrolithiasis vs. Other systems in your body can be affected when you pass a kidney stone.

Using these few overused verbs tends to make sentences longer and the meaning more obscure. This habit is not particular to non-native speakers, but if English is your second or third language, it is understandably tempting, because you have fewer verbs and therefore fewer tense and other grammar problems to worry about!

Using imagery, simile and metaphor

Complex explanations can be hard to follow, even when the language is clear, and especially if your patient is already under some stress or particularly worried about a health problem. Supporting logical, clear explanations with an image, a story – sometimes even a quick drawing – can enhance understanding, and make the information you are giving easier to remember.

ACTION POINT 11

- Try rephrasing the following medical terms in order to make them more patient friendly:

Hypertension	No signs of progression
A benign condition	Scan is reported as negative
Prognosis	Biopsy
Renal dysfunction	Bi-temporal headache
Jaundice	Partial remission

- Practise explaining a medical condition or treatment approach to a friend with a non-medical background. How much can your friend repeat back to you? How accurate is his or her account? Does he or she agree with you about which points were the most important?
- Can you think of examples where it might be useful to draw a quick picture to describe what you mean? Or use a simile: 'It's like … It's the same as …'? Or use a metaphor: 'Your heart is the engine room of your body'?

Showing empathy

We all would like to think that we are capable of showing empathy toward others when they are in particular need of our support and understanding. However, sometimes we can mistake our efforts for other kinds of response such as giving advice, telling them to cheer up, showing pity, and so on.

Showing empathy is part of the rapport you have established with your patient – sensitivity toward his or her feelings. The difficulty lies in trying to explain exactly what we mean by empathy.

We talk about three main forms of empathy: (1) cognitive empathy – we recognise what another person is feeling; (2) emotional empathy ('emotional contagion') – we actually feel what another person is feeling; (3) compassionate empathy – we want to help the person deal with his or her situation and emotions.[13] We can further define what we mean by saying that the empathetic response is non-judgemental – we make no judgement of the emotion being expressed and we don't state whether the emotion is, in our view, appropriate or proportionate to the situation. We simply acknowledge that we have seen the patient experiencing it.

Certainly, the benefits of empathetic listening are immense: it builds trust and respect; it enables the speaker to release emotions and reduces tension; it encourages surfacing of information so that listener has all the necessary information; and it creates a safe environment conducive to collaborative problem-solving.[14]

In the following scenario the patient is a 65-year-old man whose prostate biopsies show a moderately differentiated cancer. Compare the various responses from the doctor:

Patient: Cancer? No, there's got to be a mistake!

Doctor: No, it isn't a mistake. It's definitely your biopsy. [*Direct and factual response*]

or

We don't make mistakes here. [*Judgemental response*]

or

What is it that makes you say that? [*Open question*]

or

I know this is hard to believe. [*Empathetic response*][16]

Although empathy can be difficult to define, it is readily recognisable when we hear it!

ACTION POINT 12

Think about the possible responses illustrated here: direct or factual; judgemental; open question; empathetic.

Try generating different responses to the following:

- The patient presented with an atypical mycobacterium infection and has just been diagnosed as having AIDS. **Patient**: 'AIDS! Oh my God – why me?'
- A 52-year-old man has diabetes, which is well controlled. He recently lost his job. **Patient**: 'I just feel so miserable all the time.'
- The patient is a 70-year-old Gujarati-speaking woman. Before you see her, her son bursts into the room. **Son**: 'If it's cancer you are not to tell my mother.'

Is there ever a case for giving a direct/factual response? (You can find more examples like these in *Difficult Conversations in Medicine* by R Buckman.[15])

The empathetic response will often be accompanied by an open question, responding first to the patient's emotion – recognising and acknowledging the patient's feeling:

> I realise this must be a real shock for you. This is difficult to take in, isn't it?

… and again sharing your intuitive guesses in a tentative way:

> I get the feeling/I have the impression/Something tells me that/I sense that/Am I right in thinking …?

In this way you connect with the whole person rather than just the illness; you move the focus from the medical condition to how the patient is feeling about the medical condition. Once the emotion has been identified and shared, both you and your patient are 'freed' to talk openly about the medical condition and move toward a shared plan.

Last thoughts about explaining the diagnosis

Remember that 'downloading' information – however complete – can make the patient feel ignored as an individual, so think about how to present your findings. The speed at which we speak also conveys a message. Apart from possibly being difficult to follow and understand, talking very fast may convey the feeling to your patient that you are in a hurry to finish. If you have a tendency to speak quickly, remember to keep a check on this impulse – and take time to make sure that you have broken down the information into manageable chunks, with pauses so that your patient has time to assimilate the information or ask questions. This will also give you thinking time – and time to check understanding before moving on. After all, how things are explained can have a significant impact on patient adherence to the management plan.

You may find this checklist helpful at this stage of your consultation.

I have thought about …	

- What my patient knows
- What my patient wants to know
- How the medical facts balance with my patient's feelings and issues
- How much information is 'too much'?
- Giving information in manageable chunks, with pauses
- Giving explanations in a clear and concise way – avoiding jargon
- Repeating, rephrasing and summarising if necessary
- Picking up and responding to non-verbal and verbal clues
- Allowing my patient to ask questions
- Providing opportunities for my patient to say how he or she is feeling

THOUGHTS ON ... NEGOTIATING THE SHARED MANAGEMENT PLAN
Non-judgemental and inclusive communication

Carefully chosen words will make shared decision-making much easier. Be alert! Phrases like 'you should' or 'why haven't you?' immediately place the doctor in the role of some sort of critical parent, teacher or boss, with the patient as a difficult child or employee who hasn't done as he was told! Focus instead on providing options, using open-ended questions:

- Have you ever thought about ...?
- What are your thoughts about ...?
- Can you tell me more about ...?
- Would you consider trying ...?

Use inclusive language such as we, us, our, let's:

> I know you're worried about side effects, so how do you feel about starting with this medication, then let's meet again after a couple of weeks and we'll see how things are going – and we'll review our plan then if necessary. How does that sound?

Remember that even in this kind of shared decision-making, you are still the medical expert, but you are also helping your patients to take responsibility for their long-term health and well-being by encouraging a more collaborative relationship.

ACTION POINT 13

Think about the phrases provided here. Which ones sound more 'doctor centred'? Which phrases offer options?

Let's think about ...	I would advise you to ...
How about ...ing? (e.g. how about trying/taking/going ...?)	You must ...
	I'd recommend that you ...
What if we ...?	We can either ... or ...
Why don't you ...?	Have you (ever) thought about ...?
Perhaps you could ...?	You could always ...
We could consider ...	One solution/option might be to ...
I think you should ...	

(There are more practical ideas like this in *Good Practice*, a very useful book by McCullagh and Wright.[16])

ACTION POINT 14

In some cultures, if you use too much inclusive language, it is considered overly familiar. In France, for example, when your language seems familiar like this, people say, 'We didn't raise pigs together', meaning, 'keep your distance my friend!' In other cultures, it may also give the impression that you are unsure of yourself in some way, or trying to curry favour with a group to which you don't really belong.

- What is the effect of inclusive language like 'let's' in your culture? You'll have noticed that this whole chapter is written using inclusive language! How do you feel about that?
- Look at the way inclusive language is used when talking about the shared values of the NHS.

CULTURE NOTE

'Chunking' and 'signposting'

It's helpful for you, as well as your patients, to think about how you organise the information you need to give by 'signposting' for sequence and timescale. For example, first ... then ... next ... last, now, today ... next week ... tomorrow, so, moving on, thinking ahead ...

Remember that the UK cultural preference is for concise, precise, data-driven communication, with the emphasis on structure and logic. Using words and phrases to 'signpost' the delivery of information prepares the listener to take in a certain type of information.

For example:

- *sequencing information* (perhaps numbering off on your fingers): 'There are three things we need to think about ... first ... second ... last/next ... then ... so ...'
- *offering choices*: not only ... but also/both ... and .../on the one hand ... on the other hand .../there are pros and cons .../either ... or ...

If you are a non-native English speaker, you will probably find that signposting also helps you organise the information you are delivering into manageable chunks. You will naturally pause at the end of each chunk or leave a second or two of silence between parts of the diagnosis explanation, suggestions for management plan or consultation summary. This gives your patient the time to understand what is being said.

As you pause between ideas, you will find it easier to pick up on and respond to any non-verbal and verbal communication clues you notice. This will allow you to get an idea of your patient's thoughts, feelings and reactions. You may decide it's necessary to repeat, rephrase or summarise what's been said. You may want to check your patient's understanding or to reinforce one of your remarks.

Here is an example of a doctor using the chunking–signposting technique to summarise what has been agreed:

OK, so what will happen is,/first we'll get your blood test done/that will take about a week to come back/so see me again at the end of next week./Meanwhile I'll write a letter of referral to the hospital specialist./The hospital will write to you with an appointment date and time/ you should hear from them within 2 weeks./How does that sound?

Is that a 'yes' or a 'maybe'?

You can check the likelihood of your patient really agreeing – and then keeping to – any agreed plan by looking out for non-verbal communication and the use of 'dispreference markers'. Take a look at the following extract from the end of the 'negotiated plan' stage of consultation:

Doctor: So I'll leave you to sort out when you'll be seeing the practice nurse about getting help to give up smoking?

No problem	Well …	I'm sorry, but …
Yep	Er …	I'm afraid … (I won't have time this week)
Will do	Um …	
Yes, that's fine	Hmm …	Normally I would, but …
(+ bright, positive tone of voice)	(+ dropping of tone, intonation and break in eye contact)	(+ explanations or excuses)
I agree to do this	**I'm reluctant**	**I don't want to**

In this example the doctor will have noticed body language as well as the speaker's tone of voice and how he or she phrases his or her initial reaction.

When 'well' is used as a 'dispreference marker', it is usually followed by a pause, and often accompanied by a (long-winded) explanation in which the person will try to justify or explain his or her behaviour:

Doctor: How about trying to give up smoking?
Patient: Well, er … I did think about it quite seriously – I even got some of those patches you can buy, but, well, you know, it's really difficult because my partner smokes …

Here are some more examples:

Patient: Well the other doctor said … [*I don't really believe or want to believe what you're telling me.*]
Patient: Oh, well … I suppose you're right, Doctor. [*Reluctant acceptance of what you're telling me.*]

Doctor: So, do you think you could give that a try?

Patient: Mmm … Well, the thing is … [*I'm unlikely to actually do this, so I'm getting my excuses ready.*]

If you notice these kinds of dispreference markers, you'll need to probe to find out more about the patient's real concerns by picking up on tone of voice or other non-verbal clues:

- 'You sound a little unsure about this – perhaps there are some more questions you would like to ask?'
- 'I get the feeling that you're not convinced – is there anything in particular that's worrying you?'
- 'You seem doubtful – can you tell me more about that?'

Remember to look out for this sort of clue, especially when you are negotiating a plan and drawing the consultation to a close; these clues will help you to know whether the patient is really going to follow through on the plan you have 'shared' or not. Historically, at this stage of the consultation doctors tended to talk about patient 'compliance', which suggests a rather subservient doctor–patient relationship. In a patient-centred consultation the more appropriate word is concordance – agreement – but again, you'll need to use all your communication skills to decipher a passive 'polite' acceptance from a real agreement.

Being assertive and saying 'no' (politely)

There will inevitably be some occasions when you will have to refuse requests from your patients – for all sorts of good reasons, which nevertheless may not initially be acceptable to them. This kind of conversation is, of course, easier to manage when you have established a rapport with your patient. Then you will be more able to structure your explanations in such a way that you can explain and present options that will go some way toward convincing your patient and make it possible to negotiate a plan together. Nevertheless, there will be times when you will need to be firm – in order to adhere to the law, NHS protocols, your professional code of ethics, guidelines agreed within the practice where you work, and, not least, in order to manage your patient's real health needs.

Some cultures feel uncomfortable about saying 'no' or refusing a request directly. Out of politeness, or deference to the status or position of the person they are speaking to, or in order to avoid giving offence, they will prefer to say 'yes' even if they mean 'no'. If you have come from a culture with this kind of communication preference, being more assertive may feel uncomfortable at first. Even in UK culture where a degree of assertiveness is valued, even expected, some native English speakers find this hard to do – usually because they are

CULTURE NOTE

trying to avoid a potential situation of conflict. However, this is a skill that can be learnt – and it can be achieved without being aggressive or impolite.[*]

Mindfulness as a first step to assertiveness

If you think a potential situation of conflict is developing, check in with yourself and 'listen' to what your body is telling you – in other words, use your 'emotional intelligence'. Perhaps you will notice your pulse rate going up, or a churning feeling in your stomach or a strong feeling of discomfort – perhaps a strong desire to leave the situation altogether! Acknowledge your own feelings to yourself – this will then leave you 'free' to focus on being sensitive to the needs and feelings of your patient without interference (or 'noise') from your own emotions.

- 'This is a difficult situation for both of us.'
- 'I can see that you're upset.'

By acknowledging the other person's feelings you are making a start on trying to reduce the tension. That will help you to focus on how the conversation can continue. Then set out the rules and boundaries as calmly and unemotionally as you can, speaking clearly and firmly:

- 'We won't be able to sort this out while you're shouting.'
- 'I'm afraid I can't help you until you calm down so we can have a proper conversation.'

Now you can begin to de-escalate the conflict by opening up choices and finding a compromise that is workable. That does not mean giving the patient what he or she wants; indeed, doing so may do the patient harm! For example, giving a patient more methadone simply because he asks for it, or allowing a patient to stop taking essential medication to bring down her blood pressure is not kind or ethical. State the key facts calmly and clearly, but also try to acknowledge the other person's views, probe deeper to find out the reasons for the patient's demands and propose a trial alternative. As far as possible try to match what you propose with the patient's concerns:

I know you're concerned about ... so first of all what I suggest is ...

---

[*] The Centre for Clinical Interventions offers free resources for GPs on a range of topics including assertive communication – see their website (www.cci.health.wa.gov.au).

THOUGHTS ON ... BRINGING THE CONSULTATION TO A CLOSE

Toward the end of the consultation you will of course tell your patient that the consultation is coming to a close, summarise what has been said and check whether the patient has anything to add. Think about the signalling words and phrases you might use here to 'step' the conclusion?

For example:

- OK, just to recap ...
- So what we've agreed is that ...
- So let's just sum up what we've decided today ...

When checking with your patient that he or she agrees, it's useful to think about the patient's real motivation for following your advice. If you suspect that there may be something stopping the patient from following the shared plan, check that out in the final minute of the consultation by asking if he or she has anything to add. Part of your safety-netting – for example, arranging to meet the patient as soon as possible to clarify any new information if necessary – might be a response to this intuition.

USING ACRONYMS TO STRUCTURE KEY CONVERSATIONS

While an over-reliance on communication protocols or acronyms is not a good idea, using them can be helpful in organising ideas in a methodical way. Robert Buckman[15] explains in depth four strategies for breaking bad news that can be used with patients or with close relatives. Here is a brief outline of one example already discussed in Chapter 3, the SPIKES model, devised by Baile *et al.* (2000) (in Baile, Buckman and Lenzi[17]).

TABLE 4.1 SPIKES protocol for breaking bad news

S	Setting	Consider the setting for the conversation that you need to have with your patient.
P	Perception	Assess the patient's perception of his or her situation; what does the patient know, or suspect?
I	Invitation	'Invite' your patient to let you know how much information he or she wants to know about his or her current situation.
K	Knowledge	Provide the patient with the knowledge about his or her condition and the likely prognosis.
E	Emotions	Identifying which emotion is being expressed, acknowledge that feeling, show empathy and validate the patient's feelings as being normal and to be expected.
S	Summary and Strategy	Summarise the key points, honestly, clearly and concisely, and agree the most appropriate strategy for moving on.

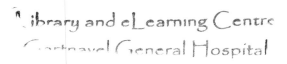

The SCORE model suggested by Robert Dilts (in Walter[18]) orders and sequences the type of information that patients typically seek regarding diagnosis, causation, treatment and prognosis – and it can help you to make sure you have covered that information.

TABLE 4.2 The SCORE model

S	Symptoms – what is initially presented
C	Causes – what has come beforehand, the reason why
O	Outcomes – what you want instead
R	Resources – what you need to bring to bear on the situation
E	Effects – the short- and the longer-term consequences

The point of these various strategies is that they provide a structure – but not a script – which can help you to decide how to approach a range of situations that will come your way in general practice.

> **ACTION POINT 15**
>
> Using the protocols provided, practise the questions you would need to ask in the consultation. If you find this way of working useful and effective, gradually add to your collection, practising the language you will need as you go.

Before we finish the chapter, here are a few thoughts about the broader aspects of your work as a GP in the UK.

LIVING AND WORKING IN THE UK
Working with patients from other cultures

CULTURE NOTE

As we said at the beginning of this chapter we have worked on the assumption that you are working with native English speakers. The reality in the GP's consulting room will probably be much more international. The key features of good interpersonal skills are of course all still valid here, but there are common issues that risk creating 'noise' when people are communicating across cultures. Here are some examples.

TABLE 4.3 Common issues that risk creating 'noise' when people are communicating across cultures

Use of English	When neither doctor nor patient are communicating in his/her first language there will be a greater tolerance of communication problems – in fact, non-native speakers tend to feel more comfortable talking with other non-native speakers However: • word meanings and word connotations are changed by cultural context • communication styles can more easily be misinterpreted (e.g. too formal or too informal) • accent and intonation – on both sides – may be harder to understand • the doctor needs to be especially attentive to his or her own use of English • interpreters – particularly if they are family members – may present a distorted view of the patient's condition, or they simply may not have sufficient language skills
Cultural norms and values about health	• Health beliefs and attitudes toward illness and disease – what is 'normal' or 'abnormal' • Cultural assumptions about the causes of illness and treatment options may be hard to talk about openly, e.g. mental health or disability • Cultural assumptions about fate and belief may determine how much effort the patient will put into his or her own treatment • Patients may also be consulting practitioners of complementary or alternative medicines
Cultural norms and values about roles and relationships	You will have to take into account: • attitudes toward gender and age • expectations about how a doctor must behave and how patients should interact with him or her • misunderstandings of legal and ethical constraints • the importance of family involvement, family structures and extended family • rituals and beliefs that accompany 'life events' – arranged marriages, pregnancy and childbirth, treatment of elders and death • extra sensitivity about sexual orientation, sexual practices and birth control • domestic violence and abuse, alcohol and drug abuse
Non-verbal communication	Awareness required about: • physical touch, and acceptable distance or closeness of 'space bubble', interpretations of body language • eye contact • expression of emotions

(continued)

Stereotyping	Do not be misled
	Cultural parameters describe only statistical realities:
	● some Indians do not believe their lives are governed by fate
	● some Germans are extremely careless about the way they organise their time
	Differences in given populations come from
	● social class
	● education
	● income level
	● professional culture
	This all may reflect in how these patients express themselves, how they perceive illness and how they make health decisions

Developing trust and mutual understanding can take time and commitment from both patient and doctor. Becoming aware of our own cultural norms, values and assumptions is the first step; we all tend to take our own culture for granted and it may be difficult for your patients to express cultural values and belief systems even in their own language. You can help them to do this.

Using interpreters in the consultation

CULTURE NOTE

You may find that your patient is unable to speak English. If you are in the fortunate position of being able to speak the home language of some of your patients, they will certainly be pleased and relieved. If not, you will need to communicate via an interpreter. Often a family member will come forward, but this is not really good practice. Apart from the lack of privacy and confidentiality for the patient, you do not know the real level of fluency of the interpreter, and therefore you cannot be sure how accurately information is being relayed. The personal relationship between patient and interpreter may also be a further source of 'noise', especially if it concerns bad news or 'taboo' subjects, which may cause embarrassment.

Best practice is to refer to specialist companies for a list of interpreters available in your area.* You could also use Language Line, which is a telephone-based interpreter service that is widely used in the NHS. Even then you will still need to make sure that sensitive issues are talked through tactfully with your patient and the interpreter at the beginning of the consultation. As always, be open about what you don't know:

> You mention that you are from Burma. I've never been there – tell me more about the culture of Burma. For example, if …, would that be considered OK?

---

* For example, see the LanguageLine Solutions website (www.languageline.co.uk)

Can you tell me a little about yourself and your family? Where do you live? Who is at home with you? Where was your family's home?

Would it be alright to ask you about …?

This may be difficult for you … the reason I need to ask is … Would you prefer to be examined by a female doctor – is that important for you?[19]

Adapting communication style

Our own individual communication style is the result of all sorts of influences: genetic inheritance; upbringing; social background; our education and training; religious beliefs; work experiences. Cultural preferences in terms of style do of course vary between the members of any particular culture, and it is useful to have some idea of our own communication style so that we are aware when, where and with whom that particular style is useful and helpful, and in what circumstances we might need to 'flex' our natural style in order to be effective.

CULTURE NOTE

If you have already taken examinations in the UK, you may have noticed differences in teaching methods and the relationship with your trainer or ES. The UK education system places value on individual autonomy, and the ability to use initiative and take responsibility for your own learning; students are encouraged to think independently and demonstrate a capacity for reflective thought through questioning, expressing original ideas, critical thinking and debate. In examination situations, you may be surprised by the way some questions require that you adopt a questioning or sceptical approach with colleagues who are senior in age or authority, or you may find that you are expected to adopt a different style when you present your answers.

No one way is necessarily better than another, but of course each culture will have its own expectations of what constitutes a 'good' and 'effective' style of thinking and communicating. When preparing for the CSA, you will be reminded that the consultation has to follow a logical structure with a line of questioning that demonstrates a clearly reasoned way of thinking. This way of processing thoughts and ideas will also be expected in many aspects of your professional communication, such as managing the structure of consultations, presenting handovers and writing case notes, reports and even emails. It may feel constraining at first, but it is possible to learn techniques that support this cultural preference – and, indeed, these are techniques that many native English speakers also have to learn in order to become more effective in their professional role.

Working as a team: the importance of 'small talk'

Having focused on the patient–doctor interaction during this chapter, we would like to share a few thoughts about your role as a member of the practice team. In general practice you will of course be working with the same people every day. Knowing this, you might be tempted to use coffee and lunch breaks to catch up with patient telephone calls, notes, or letters of referral, thinking: 'I'll catch up with the team later … this afternoon … tomorrow … some other time'. Quite apart from giving you an opportunity to have a break and a change of scene, your team is part of your support network, and you are part of theirs, so it's important to play your part in building and maintaining the team.

Remember that making small talk, like all communication, is as much about listening and asking questions – showing that we are interested in the other person – as it is about talking. As a general principle, just keep your eyes and ears open and notice the 'cultural norms and behaviours' in your workplace.

ACTION POINT 16

- Which topics of conversation would be acceptable in your home culture?
- Observe what people talk about in your work practice. Are you surprised or not? Do you find it easy to join in? If not, what might make it easier?

Planning the next steps

In this chapter we have looked at communication: how it works and why it sometimes breaks down, the impact of culture on communication, language choices for patient-centred consultations, aspects of non-verbal communication, ways of picking up on patient cues, and some things to look out for when using English in your professional role in the UK. You have also been invited to reflect on your own preferred communication style and explore ways of enhancing your awareness of communication strategies through the Action Points. In conclusion, here are a few closing remarks …

For many of the doctors we meet – most of whom already have a very good level of English – the complexity of using English in a professional context is still a challenge, particularly when under pressure because of time constraints, heavy work schedule, additional training commitments and general fatigue. As we have seen, being an effective communicator requires extensive language skills, but also a knowledge and understanding of the cultural context of that language. Think about how you will address this language or culture dimension to your work.

It's tempting to postpone this initiative – all doctors have huge pressures on their time and many even feel guilty about 'leisure' reading when they feel they ought to be keeping up to date with the latest research in their field. If it helps, think about this as a career investment – as part of your long-term career development plan.

On the other hand, you can think of this as an essential part of your own work–life balance – the 'downtime' that will help you to be fully present for your patients when you are with them – and a fully 'rounded' person with a life of your own when you are not. Whatever you choose to do to extend and enhance your English skills, make it something painless, enjoyable and relaxing – and as much as possible outside the medical setting. Here are some ideas to get you going.

TABLE 4.4 Ideas for enhancing interpersonal communication skills

Outside work	✓	At work	✓
What can I read/listen to/do/that will give me a feeling for popular culture? ● Read the occasional tabloid newspaper such as the Daily Mail or the Express ● Go along to local events and festivals ● Listen to local radio		How can I increase my easy-going social contact with colleagues? ● Coffee room ● Lunching with a partner ● Going to holiday parties and events	
How can I find out what makes the British laugh? ● Watch TV/listen to radio – particularly 'stand-up' comedians and satirical news programmes ● Notice the interactions between people in shops, trains, cafes, etc.		How can I get organised to attend multidisciplinary team meetings and case conferences? Which colleagues would I feel comfortable about asking for a debrief?	
What could I do to improve my pronunciation and intonation? ● Join a choir? ● Join an amateur dramatics group? ● Practice by repeating phrases from TV or radio		Which joint surgeries can I get involved in so that I can observe more experienced colleagues? How do I find out about setting this up?	
What kind of community association could I get involved in that would help me to understand the British better? ● Parent school groups? ● Charity organisations and events? ● Sports clubs and associations?		Which CPD opportunities are happening right now that might interest me?	✓
Does my church or religious institution have a group or association where I could get to know local people in my community?		Where can I attend – or how can I set up – an Action Learning Set with colleagues to talk through shared experiences and challenges?	

TOP TIPS FOR YOUR ACTION PLAN

Set yourself realistic weekly targets for enhancing your interpersonal communication skills and plan time to allow you to achieve them.

If you have family with you, this is a great opportunity to integrate your language and culture discovery activities with family life – and compare your experiences and achievements.

Think about keeping a journal – or a family log – to celebrate your achievements as you settle into your new life.

CONCLUDING THOUGHTS

Most of us feel that it's important that we are at some level known and appreciated by those we work and live with – partners, family, friends, colleagues and patients. We want to be valued and acknowledged for the work we do – as well as for the people we are. Naturally this takes time and not all of our interactions will allow time for these relationships to develop fully – indeed, it is not always appropriate or necessary that they should. Nevertheless, as human beings and social animals the longing is still there.

Occasionally we may be surprised by the inaccuracy (or the accuracy!) of the way we are seen and interpreted. When we are caught in the maelstrom of our working lives, sometimes physically and mentally exhausted, it can be easy to feel that we are not being 'seen' or valued for who we are and what we do. Living and working in another culture also means adjusting on several levels and can generate a range of reactions and unexpected emotions. You may sometimes feel isolated or doubt your professional competencies. You may even feel resentful about having to adapt your usual behaviour or uncomfortable about the way this makes you feel about yourself. These feelings can cause anxiety, stress, even guilt, as well as extreme fatigue.

Remember to keep your channels of communication open and try to remain receptive to help which is available from your support network of work colleagues and friends. As you become immersed in your new working environment and further enhance your language skills, you will notice that you are able to observe the culture from the inside as well as the outside. You will find it easier to flex your communication style and adjust to the cultural shift you are making – national, organisational and professional – while still remaining true to your authentic self. I hope that the journey we have started here will be helpful to you as you make your own unique and excellent contribution to the NHS.

Some patients, though conscious that their condition is perilous, recover their health simply through their contentment with the goodness of the physician.

Hippocrates, 400 BC

REFERENCES

1. Goleman D. *Social Intelligence*. Croydon: Arrow Books; 2006.
2. Hargie O. *Skilled Interpersonal Communication: research, theory and practice*. 5th ed. Hove: Routledge; 2011.
3. Tate P. *The Doctor's Communication Handbook*. 5th ed. Oxford: Radcliffe Publishing; 2010.
4. Lewis RD. *When Cultures Collide: leading across cultures*. 3rd revised ed. London; Nicholas Brealey Publishing; 2005.
5. Korsch BM, Negrete VF. Doctor-patient communication. *Sci Am.*1972; **227**(2): 66–74.
6. Fox K. *Watching the English: the hidden rules of English behaviour*. St Ives: Hodder & Stoughton; 2005.
7. Guirdham M. *Communicating Across Cultures at Work*. 2nd ed. Basingstoke: Palgrave Macmillan; 2005.
8. Mehrabian A. *Non-Verbal Communication*. Piscataway, NJ: Aldine Transaction; 2007.
9. Ekman P. *Emotions Revealed*. London: Phoenix; 2004.
10. Rogers C. *On Becoming a Person*. New ed. London: Constable & Robinson; 2004.
11. Beckman HB, Frankel RM. The effect of physician behaviour on the collection of data. *Ann Intern Med.* 1984; **101**(5): 692–6.
12. Neighbour R. *The Inner Consultation*. Oxford: Radcliffe Publishing; 2005.
13. Preston SD, de Waal FB. Empathy: its ultimate and proximate bases. *Behav Brain Sci.* 2002; **25**(1): 1–20.
14. Salem R. *Empathic Listening*. Boulder, CO: Beyond Intractability – Conflict Research Consortium, University of Colorado; 2003. Available at: www.beyondintractability.org/essay/empathic-listening (accessed 10 October 2013).
15. Buckman R. *Difficult Conversations in Medicine*. Baltimore, MD: John Hopkins University Press; 2010.
16. McCullagh M, Wright R. *Good Practice: communication skills in English for the medical practitioner*. Cambridge: Cambridge University Press; 2008.
17. Baile WF, Buckman R, Lenzi R, *et al*. SPIKES—a six-step protocol for delivering bad news: application to the patient with cancer. *Oncologist*. 2000; **5**(4): 302–11.
18. Walter L. *Consulting with NLP*. Oxford: Radcliffe Medical Press; 2002.
19. Silverman J, Kurtz S, Draper J. *Skills for Communicating with Patients*. Oxford: Radcliffe Publishing; 2005.

CHAPTER 5

Succeeding at assessment

This chapter concentrates on trying to give you some guidance to help you jump through the hoops* that stand between you and becoming a fully fledged† GP. To become a GP in the UK these hoops are encapsulated within the MRCGP exam. The MRCGP is an assessment in three parts and tests all aspects of general practice. The three parts are as follows:

1. Applied Knowledge Test (or AKT), which is a knowledge-based multiple-choice answer paper.
2. Clinical Skills Assessment (or CSA), which is effectively a simulated surgery, which tests both your ability to apply your clinical knowledge to practical situations and your consulting ability.
3. Workplace-based assessment (or WPBA), which is based upon your e-portfolio and performance within actual GP practice.

Inevitably, people concentrate more on the exam-based components of the assessment, but it is important to remember that all three are in fact equally important. While more unusual, it is entirely possible to pass both your AKT and CSA and yet still not be signed up for your CCT because of your performance in the WPBA component.

All of these components are based on the RCGP curriculum, so it makes sense to ensure that you are familiar with this. Inevitably, this is a large document to get to grips with,‡ but a good place to start would be reading the first curriculum statement, 'Being a General Practitioner'.[1] It is also useful to look at a specific clinical area if you are about to undertake a particular specialty in secondary care. You could even consider sharing this with your CS, as it will

---

Phrase notes

* 'jump through hoops' – to do a lot of extra things so that you have or do something you want

† 'fully fledged' – of full status (i.e. fully qualified as a GP)

‡ 'get to grips with' – to begin to deal with someone or something difficult or challenging in a sensible way

help him or her to understand what your educational needs might be from a primary care perspective.

ACTION POINT 1

Read 'Being a General Practitioner' (available at: www.rcgp.org.uk/gp-training-and-exams/gp-curriculum-overview.aspx).

Going into the detail of the RCGP curriculum is beyond the scope of this book. It is all available, and updated, on the RCGP website.[2] To make it more manageable, however, you might like to check out one of the many guides to the MRCGP exam that are available, or at least look at *The Condensed Curriculum Guide*.[3]

It is also probably worth thinking about what aspects of your work as a GP each component is designed to test, as this may help you to focus your preparation better. This can be looked at with respect to Miller's pyramid (*see* Figure 5.1).[4]

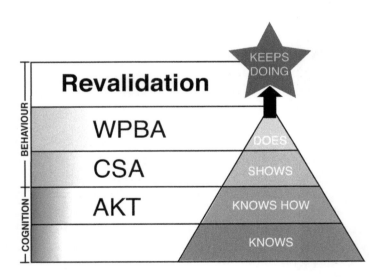

FIGURE 5.1 Miller's pyramid in relation to the Membership of the Royal College of General Practitioners exam

APPLIED KNOWLEDGE TEST

You can apply to take your AKT at any point from your second year of training (St2) onwards. It consists of 200 machine-marked questions – approximately 80% will be on clinical medicine, 10% on critical appraisal and 10% on health informatics. The test is not negatively marked.

SOMETHING TO THINK ABOUT

Because part of the AKT tests aspects of the business and management side of general practice, does it make sense to sit it before you have experienced a general practice placement?

It takes place at approximately 150 venues (spread across the country) that are usually used for the theory component of the UK driving assessment. You can find details of the possible venues online (www.pearsonvue.com/rcgp). The exam is held three times a year, usually at the end of January, the end of April and the end of October, with the choice of a morning or afternoon session each time. Bookings for the exam usually open in the second week of the preceding month – that is, bookings for October usually open toward the beginning of September.

The RCGP has found that OMGs particularly seem to struggle with the less clinical aspects of knowledge that are needed, such as the health informatics and critical appraisal questions. This may in part be due to a lack of information as to the content that features in these aspects of the exam. So recently the RCGP have produced an AKT content guide,[5] which goes into more detail of exactly what you can expect the exam to cover. The content guide also covers some of the clinical curriculum areas, although trying to look at the entire guide in one sitting might well be overwhelming. There is a good introduction as to how to use the guide most effectively, which is worth reading first rather than diving straight in.[*]

Being in a general practice setting will also help you to understand some of these less clinical aspects of the exam, so it is probably worth waiting until you have been in primary care for at least 3–6 months before applying to sit it. You also need to be aware that you will have a maximum of four attempts at passing your AKT, so it makes sense to ensure that you make the most of each of these. Although obviously we hope it won't take you four goes!

ACTION POINT 2

- Check out the AKT content guide[†]
- Consider using Section 3 (Administrative, Ethical and Regulatory Frameworks) to set some learning objectives for a tutorial with your practice manager

---

Phrase notes

* 'to dive straight in' – to start something enthusiastically without first thinking about it
† AKT content guide can be found at www.rcgp.org.uk/gp-training-and-exams/mrcgp-exam-overview/mrcgp-applied-knowledge-test-akt.aspx#content

Practical things to consider

For the most up-to-date information, please ensure that you look at the latest guidance regarding exams on the RCGP website.

- **Check online* for when bookings open for your chosen sitting and book early.** If you want to take your test at a popular location, ensure you book early, as these centres book up quickly – otherwise you may find yourself adding a significant travelling distance to your stress.
- **Ensure you take the appropriate identification documents with you on the day to the test centre.** You need to take with you two forms of identification – one containing your name, address and a photo (such as a current passport or a UK photo card driving licence) and one containing your name and signature, such as a credit card. These must be in the name with which you are registered with the RCGP; if the two names are different (e.g. one is in your maiden name and one in your married name), then you must also take an official document that links the two. It has been known for people not to be allowed to sit the exam because they have not had the appropriate documentation. If you are unsure about what you need to take to reconcile two different names, then contact the Exams department at RCGP – they will be able to advise you further.

I couldn't believe that they wouldn't let me sit the exam because I didn't have the right I.D. That's a lesson I won't forget!

Maria

- **Answer *all* the questions.** The AKT is not negatively marked, so you have nothing to lose by guessing if you are not sure of an answer. Often you will be able to rule out one or two of the possible answers immediately and this significantly increases the odds of getting the answer right.
- **Don't keep reviewing your answers.** Research suggests that your first answer is the one that is most likely to be the right one, so unless you are absolutely certain that you are wrong, don't keep reviewing and changing your answers.
- **Disclose in advance any specific learning difficulties that may affect your performance.** The AKT is quite a time-pressured test for anyone – 200 questions in 3 hours is a mean duration of 54 seconds per question. If you are answering questions in your second language, then it is even more likely to be time-pressured for you. Add in a specific learning difficulty, such as dyslexia, and it is likely that you will run into difficulties with time management. Do not be embarrassed to admit this, as you will then be given extra time to complete the test, which may make all the difference between success and failure. In order to access this additional time you will need to

---

* www.rcgp.org.uk/gp-training-and-exams/mrcgp-exam-overview/mrcgp-applied-knowledge-test-akt.aspx

explain your situation to the RCGP (when you apply to sit the exam) and they will require a report from an educational psychologist to confirm this. If you suspect this may be true but you have never been formally tested, then talk to your deanery in good time and they may be able to help you access appropriate testing (this means not waiting until you have repeatedly failed the exam). If you do get offered extra time then you will have to sit the exam in one of the afternoon sittings. If your deanery does not have easy access to dyslexia testing there are a number of online tools that you could try that might help you to decide whether it is worth exploring further. For example, you could check out Spot your Potential (www.spot-your-potential.com/index.htm) or the British Dyslexia Association website (www.bdadyslexia.org.uk). It is worth remembering, however, that these tools are designed for people whose native tongue is English and they may not be as accurate, with a tendency toward over-diagnosis, in individuals for whom English is a second language.

I wish someone had told me about dyslexia earlier. Maybe then it wouldn't have taken me three goes. And think how much money I'd have saved!

Madhavi

Preparing for the AKT

- **Start early and don't underestimate the difficulty of the exam.** The AKT is not an easy exam, so you will need to put some effort into passing it! It is, however, based on what you do everyday, as it is about the knowledge that underpins your clinical practice. If you can cope with patients coming in at regular intervals with a wide spectrum of clinical conditions, then dealing with multiple-choice questions across a similar breadth should be achievable.

I underestimated the preparations for AKT and didn't pass initially but the second time I was determined to pass so I studied hard and I passed.

Gloria

- **Practise your maths.** Calculators are currently not allowed in the AKT (although there are plans for this to change), but there will be some questions that involve calculations. For some people these are difficult (and time-consuming) because of lack of practice, but these are easy marks so it makes sense to refresh your mental arithmetic. The questions will be set with user-friendly figures that are easy to use for the calculations, so if your answer comes up with an obscure fraction it is quite likely to be wrong.
- **Look at the sample questions online (www.rcgp.org.uk) and in *InnovAiT*.** The RCGP provide free sample questions, both on their website and in the

journal *InnovAiT*. It makes sense to look at these sources, as they will give you an idea of the types of question structure that are used. You can also be certain that they will be of the right level of difficulty, as the AKT examiners often write them. This can then help you to decide whether other commercially available questions are pitched correctly. It may also be worth asking your colleagues who have already sat the exam which websites and books they found useful in their preparation.

- **Look at the AKT report on the RCGP website.** This report highlights the areas in which candidates have scored poorly in previous exam sittings. Think about it – it is telling you the topics that will come up and so are worth revising! There is also the new AKT content guide[5] to review, as discussed earlier.

- **Use your patients as an educational resource.** The AKT is designed to test the knowledge base that underpins your competence as an independent GP in the UK. So using the unmet needs of your patients to highlight your educational needs (patients' unmet needs, or PUNs, and doctors' educational needs, or DENs) is one of the best tools for establishing gaps in your knowledge that need filling! This also provides good evidence for the WPBA component of your training.

- **Read the *British National Formulary* (BNF).** Review the first section of the *BNF*, which concentrates on the principles of prescribing. Also familiarise yourself with the main drug classes and recognised side effects. Which ones should you look at? Start with the ones that are commonly prescribed in general practice. Think about issues that commonly come up as clinical audits – for example, what regular monitoring bloods do individuals with rheumatoid arthritis need if they are on disease modifying therapy? Becoming familiar with the *BNF* will also be useful preparation for your CSA.

- **Consider a broad-based update course.** GP update courses can be an excellent way of getting a crash course in the latest clinical knowledge and evidence. It can also help to highlight clinical areas where your knowledge base is weak and so where you need to concentrate on. There are two main national providers of such courses – GP Update and NB Medical Education – and your deanery may offer subsidised places at one or other of them. If you do choose to go on such a course, ensure you schedule it so that you have enough time to revise any areas of learning need that it helps you to identify, rather than sending you into a blind panic about how little you think you know.

- **Remember the organisational and health informatics questions.** The clinical aspect of the exam is very broad, which can make knowing what to revise difficult. In contrast, health informatics is much more constrained and so easier to target. Try brainstorming the possible subject areas that might come up with some of your colleagues and then share out the work of providing an up-to-date accurate summary of the information. Suggestions might be political hot topics such as GP commissioning, death certification, access to medical records and data protection and driving regulations. Also check out the new AKT content guide,[5] which clearly lays out the areas that you can expect this section of questions to cover.

I didn't really understand much about the NHS system, as most of my life was spent in Africa.

Gloria

- **Remember the critical appraisal questions.** These questions are not difficult so they can provide you with easy marks, and remember one question really can make all the difference between success and failure. If you find statistics difficult, then find a course that addresses it or encourage your GP training PDs to put one on for you. Also, as with all adult learning, don't be ashamed to say that you don't understand; one of the tests of a good teacher is the teacher's ability to adapt his or her session to fulfil the needs of different levels of learners.

ACTION POINT 3

Find out what preparation courses my deanery offers for the AKT – for example, some deaneries offer subsidised places at GP Update or NB Medical Education courses.

Other resources to consider exploring:
- AKT preparation guide from the Bradford Vocational Training Scheme (www. bradfordvts.co.uk/MRCGP/akt.htm)
- *How to Revise for the AKT – A Guide for AiTs* (http://bromleygptp.org/ Other%20documents/AKT_how%20to%20revise.htm)
- Houghton M, Charlton R. *Applied Knowledge Test – Practice Questions and Answers CD.* RCGP: London; 2013 (available from the RCGP bookshop).

CLINICAL SKILLS ASSESSMENT

The CSA is a simulated surgery of 13 10-minute GP consultations held at the RCGP headquarters at 30 Euston Square, London, which is taken during your final (St3) year of training. All of the cases contain material that is covered within the GP curriculum and are aspects of medicine that you might come across in everyday clinical practice. So it is like a normal GP surgery, although admittedly it is the surgery from hell that you hope doesn't happen too often! Some of the cases have a real clinical focus whereas others might have more of an ethical dimension to them. There will also be consultations where you will have to demonstrate your proficiency at clinical examination and use of diagnostic instruments, and also your ability to prescribe safely. A different examiner will mark each of your cases, so you will have 13 different people observing your consulting behaviour. They mark each case according to three separate domains: (1) data gathering, technical and assessment skills, (2) clinical management and (3) interpersonal skills. Each domain carries the same number of marks, which are then used to contribute to your final mark, with each case carrying equal weight.

At present the CSA occurs three times a year, in November, February and May. You book for the exam online but, unlike the AKT, there is no longer any advantage in booking early, as the exam sessions are randomly allocated once the booking window has closed. The booking windows are in September, December and March. You cannot choose a specific date for your exam, but if there are dates that would be impossible for you to attend then you can specify these at the time of booking. There are however plans to start running the CSA more regularly throughout the year, such as one week in each month. Like the AKT, you are allowed to attempt the exam a maximum of four times.

You can find the most up-to-date and detailed information online.*

The CSA component is the part of the MRCGP exam that most individuals who qualified abroad fear most. It would seem that this is probably well founded, as the statistics speak for themselves.[6,7]

TABLE 5.1 Fail rates of MRCGP first attempts at AKT and CSA, 2010–11[7]

Assessment	UK graduates	OMGs	Ratio (OMG:UK graduates)
AKT	13.4%	45.6%	3.4:1
CSA	8.2%	59.2%	7.2:1

I shared a lift to London with three of my colleagues. We were all Asian males who graduated overseas. I looked round the car and thought that at least one of us was going to fail. I hoped, and prayed, that it wouldn't be me!

Sidhu

The RCGP has been doing a considerable amount of research[8–10] to try to ensure that the exam is not inherently biased against OMGs. Other postgraduate exams also show a similar pattern of pass rate discrepancy.[11] The MRCGP exam has recently been the subject of a judicial review, which found in favour of the RCGP, and judged the CSA to be lawful and fair.

So why is there such a difference in the exam results of different candidates? Well, the exam tests your competence to be a UK general practitioner and that culture of consulting may vary widely from that experienced in your home country. That doesn't mean that we, the British, are right and you are wrong. It

---

* See www.rcgp.org.uk/gp-training-and-exams/mrcgp-exam-overview/mrcgp-clinical-skills-assessment-csa.aspx

simply means that, in this country, patients have come to expect certain things and, if you don't know and respect that, then you will be like a fish out of water.* And that's before you take into account any language issues …

> Compared to UK in India consultations are different. Patients expect you to know everything and you cannot look in books, like the BNF, or offer to get back to them with more information.
>
> In India it is more doctor led and patients accept your management. There is no negotiation on the plan.
>
> Rashmi

So is it possible to reverse the trend? Yes, it most definitely is! One of the Oxford OMGs recently went from failing the CSA to improving his mark by over 30 marks to become the highest-scoring candidate in the deanery. Similarly, other areas are reporting success among their OMGs. We hope that this book, and particularly Chapter 4 on language and communication skills, will help you to be one of the success stories too.

Tips for failure: that is, things to *avoid*

- **Don't be pressurised into sitting the exam before you are ready!** The CSA is designed to ensure that your consulting ability is of the level needed to be an independent practitioner in the UK. That means that it is a test of your competence at the level expected at the *end* of your training. So why sit it too early? Don't bow to the peer pressure of your fellow St3s or even your GP training PDs – other people may well be ready before you if they don't face similar challenges. As an OMG, your starting line is further back than that of someone who has been continually immersed in the British way of practising medicine. So even if you make progress at the same rate as them, it will still take you longer to reach the same point that is the summative level of the CSA.

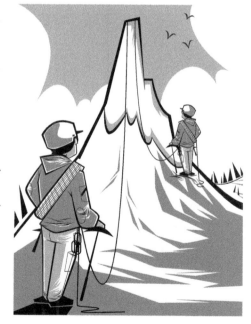

Phrase notes
* 'fish out of water' – being in a behavioural state outside your comfort zone

When I reflect back and watch a local graduate doing the consultation, I can see the difference. I have to raise my standards, after all the exam circumstances are the same for everyone, maybe my starting point is different.

Shaneil

- **Don't spend all your money on going on lots of different courses!** This tip seems rather ironic given that you have spent good money on this book! However, the cost of this is nothing compared with what you could spend going on a multitude of different courses. For most people that is not a good idea, as it will just result in more and more confusion as you search for that elusive magic answer that really doesn't exist. So should you go on any courses at all? We think going on one course is probably a good idea, so check out what your deanery offers. Find out whether the course they offer is run by actual CSA assessors or not, as this will give you a good idea as to whether the feedback you get is at the right level. Courses run by GP trainers seem to provide less critical feedback for those participating, which can lead to falsely high expectations and miss the opportunity to identify those areas that need further development.

  The only other course we would suggest that you properly consider is one based at the examination centre itself. These are usually run by the RCGP and can be helpful, especially if you are someone who gets particularly nervous in unfamiliar environments. It will give you a chance to try out the transport arrangements and get a sneaky peek* at the venue before the real thing. Sometimes the RCGP runs case piloting events at the exam centre which can be a useful educational opportunity, although places often become available with relatively short notice and are always snapped up really quickly. Obviously if you are unfortunate enough to have failed the exam at your first attempt and your deanery offers a course, which is often free of charge, targeted specifically at this group, then go on it. After all why would you look a gift horse in the mouth?† The RCGP has also recently started offering specific courses run by examiners that are only accessible to those who have previously failed the exam and these would be worth exploring if you find yourself in this situation.

I found the CSA course run by the RCGP and our deanery very helpful.

Gloria

Phrase notes

* 'sneaky peek' – an opportunity to see something before it is officially available

† 'why would you look a gift horse in the mouth' – why would you not be grateful for something that is offered to you

I think instead of going on lots of CSA courses IMGs could do language polishing.

Shahida

- **Don't buy a new suit!** The CSA is expensive enough without wasting money on clothes that you won't wear again. And trust us, the examiners' beady eyes will notice if you leave the label attached so that you can return it later (and yes, I (MF) have seen that)! Don't listen to those who say that a conservative navy or black suit will enhance your likelihood of success – examiners really aren't that shallow. You do need to be smart but you also need to be comfortable. After all, you haven't been wearing torn, paint-splattered jeans to work for the past 3 years (at least we hope you haven't!). Wear something familiar that you would wear to work, provided it is not too sexy or flashy. The more you can make the CSA seem like an ordinary morning surgery (admittedly, the surgery from hell!) rather than a high-pressure exam, the more likely you are to succeed. You might also like to think about some layers so that you can adjust your clothing to account for the ambient temperature, which can be variable. If you are concerned about what is appropriate to wear there is now a dress code that can be found on the RCGP website,[12] which may be worth you exploring for more information.

You need to find people who can give you good advice. So many IMGs simply believe the crap they are told.

Rakesh

- **Don't stress yourself out with travelling.** We know that hotels in London are expensive, but an overnight stay in the local Premier Inn (other budget chains are available!) is considerably less than the cost of resitting the exam if the rail network or airline lets you down and you arrive late and stressed, or even miss it altogether. You could even incorporate some London culture into your trip – we are not suggesting going out clubbing until early morning the day before, but you could fit in an art gallery, theatre performance or similar, depending on your personal preference. Particularly if this is a very high-stakes* exam, such as your final-allowed attempt, it is important to reduce your stress as much as possible. For we are sure you are all familiar with the stress/burnout curve, where a small amount of stress may improve your performance but too much stress will significantly deteriorate it.
- **Don't try to be someone else!** We are all individuals and so we all consult in different ways. The hole that OMGs sometimes fall into is trying to be someone else. That is difficult at the best of times, but even harder in the stress of an exam. It is often when OMGs are trying to be someone else that

---

Phrase notes
* 'high-stakes' – there is a lot to lose

they run into difficulties; dropping in so-called rote questions such as: 'What will you tell your wife when you get home?' at inappropriate points. Think about how often, or not, you have used such phrases in your everyday consulting. Asking such questions when the patient has already told you the answer also just serves to demonstrate that you are not listening properly. It may be that when observing your colleagues you find that they seem to use phrases that work really well for them. Sometimes incorporating these into your own style works well. Sometimes, however, what works for someone else is completely at odds with who you are. For example, one of my colleagues often uses metaphors relating to golf within the context of consultations, which for me (MF) would be disastrous, as I know nothing at all about golf. Using metaphors that are outside of your experience is likely to be problematic for anyone. Also, sometimes simply having the knowledge about a situation is very different from having experiential understanding of it, and this can influence how comfortable you feel addressing some issues within the consultation. For example, we may be able to explore the constraints of Ramadan for a patient with diabetes but we would find it hard to empathise completely with how this feels and its true effect on daily life.

Also, if there is a case, such as a request for a termination of pregnancy, that goes against your moral or religious beliefs, don't change your behaviour just because it is an exam. Yes, you have obligations under the GMC good medical practice[13] to ensure that the patient is able to access care appropriately and you should be able to demonstrate this. However, you do not have to compromise your beliefs for the sake of an exam, and doing so is likely to backfire, as your discomfort will become self-evident. It is a myth that you will fail for respecting your beliefs; if you fail such a case it will be because of how you communicated with the patient and helped to facilitate an alternative way of accessing care.

You will find lots more information about language, culture and consulting throughout this book. We hope that you will find it a useful starting point for thinking through these aspects.

- **Don't fall into the trap of over- or under-familiarity.** Even down to practice level you may find that there is considerable variation in how doctors address patients and patients are encouraged to address doctors. There may also be variation depending on the age of the patient, the difference in age between the doctor and the patient, the gender of either, prior knowledge of each other, social class and cultural backgrounds. There are risks associated with both over- and under-familiarity. Sometimes individuals who have previously been given feedback that they are 'too doctor centred' have concluded that overfamiliarity is a way of compensating for that. However, names are a potential minefield* – for example, if you were to call me

---

Phrase notes
* 'potential minefield' – a situation that has many potential hazards or dangers

Amanda (MF) then that would presume a level of familiarity that I have not agreed to, as anyone who knows me realises I am known as Mandy. Conversely, if you called me Mrs Fry I would be looking around for my mother! Sometimes using a patient's full name, such as Richard Mumford, can be a good way of avoiding this trap, at least initially.

- **Don't try to be too nice.** Sometimes people think that being patient centred means agreeing to whatever the patient wants, particularly if you have previously been given feedback that you have a tendency to be doctor centred. For example, there may well be patients who would prefer not to be referred to hospital but for whom a timely referral would be the most appropriate clinical action. Delaying the 2-week referral for an older woman with a breast lump so she can go on holiday for 6 weeks may make her happier in the short term, but it certainly won't help in the longer term if she turns out to have breast cancer. It is a myth that passing your CSA just involves saying 'yes' to whatever the patient requests – this may make you popular with the role player but they are not the ones marking your consultation! You need to counterbalance good interpersonal skills with sound clinical judgement. Simply being nice is not enough.

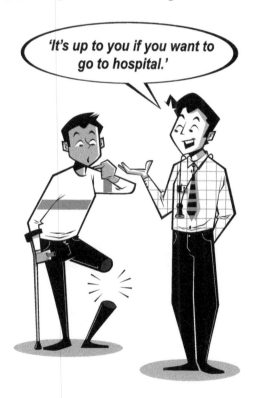

'It's up to you if you want to go to hospital.'

- **Don't always assume that there is a hidden agenda.** Just like in practice, some patients will come with a hidden agenda – for example, the patient with a headache who is worried about a brain tumour because her friend died last year after a delay in diagnosis. However, they will not *all* come with such issues. You need to ask them what their ideas, concerns and expectations are, but don't keep on and on at it. If you continually press the patient to explain why he or she has come, and what he or she thinks is going on, then the patient may even start to feel guilty for not having thought about it in more depth. This can then really affect the rest of the consultation, as you lose rapport with the patient. Also, if the patient has already told you his or her concerns don't then ask again! This just makes it look like you weren't listening the first time. Of course you could just check that there isn't anything else: 'I know that you've told me that you are worried about a brain tumour [i.e. prove you were listening!], but I wondered if there was anything else that had been going through your mind?' If they say no, leave it alone; it is not just with sex that no really means no! Sometimes rather than thinking about ideas, concerns and expectations, which can really be quite medical, it can be better to think about thoughts, worries and hopes.

- **Don't treat the exam as a tick-box exercise.** The CSA is not designed as a tick-box exercise. Rather than trying to cover every aspect in every consultation, concentrate on what is important. The skill you need to demonstrate is being able to take a *focused* history and examination. If you think about your usual practice in your surgery, you do not go over every aspect in every case. Also remember that the feedback statements are just that. They are designed to give you some constructive advice as to the areas in which you could improve in future. They are not a marking schedule and so they will not all carry equal weight in every consultation. The examiners will only turn to them *after* they have marked the case. On the RCGP website there are detailed suggestions for improvements relating to each of the feedback statements,[14] so it is worth looking at these in detail. These are a particularly valuable resource if you find that there are recurring themes from multiple consultations, such as from a previous failed attempt at the CSA.
- **Don't share options artificially.** Being patient centred is important, but sometimes there are no options to share. The patient who you suspect is having a myocardial infarction doesn't really get to choose whether or not he or she would like to go to hospital, even if the patient only believes it to be indigestion. In this sort of case you can demonstrate your patient centredness in other ways, such as taking on board the patient's anxiety, offering to phone his wife or similar, and ensuring that you share your concerns with them sensitively. If there are options to share then don't just list them but ensure that the patient has sufficient information about each one to be able to make an informed choice. Sometimes dividing the options into subgroups can help with this; for example, a woman presenting with period pain could be initially offered hormonal or non-hormonal methods to consider, *provided* that you have explained both of these options properly.

Also, if there is genuine choice within a consultation, with several options being of similar clinical value, make sure you don't bias a patient toward a particular option when you describe it to him or her.

- **Don't always assume that the examiner will give you the examination findings.** About a third of CSA cases are designed to test your ability to undertake one or more aspects of clinical examination. So explaining what you would go on to do is simply wasting time – just get on and do it! That doesn't mean that you shouldn't explain to the patient what you are about to do and gain their consent but, again, think about what you would do in everyday practice. Usually we would be explaining to the patient as we proceed with the examination. So it would be appropriate to do the same within the context of your CSA. Otherwise you are simply wasting valuable time waiting for the examiner to intervene while the examiner is waiting for you to get on with it.

  Clinical examinations should also be focused appropriately. Offering to examine the entire nervous system (unless really indicated by the clinical scenario) does not gain you extra marks for thoroughness; it gives the impression that you have no idea what you are looking for. It may also waste a huge amount of time if the examiner lets you do it.

  While it is true that you are very unlikely to be expected to undertake an intimate examination on a role player, it is entirely possible that there may be a mannequin or model for these situations. Also remember that good practice would mean that you should offer a chaperone when considering such examinations. It is true that the role player will not have true clinical signs (unlike some other postgraduate exams), but your examination technique will be judged against the criteria that you are sufficiently competent such that, if there were physical signs present, you would have been able to elicit them.

- **Don't hang on to previous cases.** So Mrs Jones has left and you realise that you have absolutely no idea what was wrong with her. In fact maybe you even realised that halfway through the consultation! Obviously that is not ideal, but the marking schedule means that each case is an opportunity to collect marks. You no longer pass or fail on the number of cases that you complete successfully but on a combined mark from all 13 cases. So use all the cases, even the ones that have gone badly, as an opportunity to gain marks. And once Mrs Jones has left, put her behind you and move on – don't waste time worrying about how badly you have done.

So if those are the top things to avoid, what should you do to prepare instead? Well, that is simple – honestly, it really is. The answer is *practise, practise and practise!*

BUT FIRST, SOME LIGHT RELIEF ...

Check out this YouTube video:

'Ice Ice Baby (how to pass CSA)'
www.youtube.com/watch?v=NawlXnyOJDY

Some of it really is very close to the mark!

So how should you practise? The obvious place to start is in your surgery, by seeing lots of patients. After all, that is what the CSA is designed to test: how you consult in practice. It is by practising that you become a fluent consulter, able to adjust your style in response to the patient's contribution.

BUT FIRST YOU NEED TO CONSOLIDATE YOUR CLINICAL KNOWLEDGE ...

Another YouTube video for you to watch!

'Test Your Awareness: Do the Test'
www.youtube.com/watch?v=Ahg6qcgoay4

If you have to concentrate too hard on one aspect of the consultation (such as core clinical knowledge) then it is easy to miss other aspects (such as patient cues). So make sure that the aspect you can control, your clinical knowledge, is at your fingertips, as then you can concentrate on your consulting behaviour and communication skills.

SOME IDEAS TO HELP YOU PRACTISE

- Whenever you give an information leaflet to a patient, print out a copy for yourself. This will help you to develop your explanations for patients (you won't get away with saying, 'Why don't you read this leaflet?' in your CSA). It may also help to highlight management options that you might not have been aware of and will show you any holes in your clinical knowledge.

ACTION POINT 4

- Log into www.patient.co.uk when you log on in the morning. This will give you prompt, easy access to good-quality patient information leaflets for patients.
- Also, register for www.gpnotebook.co.uk – then you can easily access this and even track your learning for your e-portfolio. This will highlight common clinical areas for you to focus on.

- **Video yourself consulting.** Ideally you could then watch the videos with your trainer, but just reviewing them yourself can help to identify the areas that you need to develop. It can also help you to notice any particular strategies that you use that are effective, or any habits that are annoying.

ACTION POINT 5

Ensure that you have at least one video surgery each week. Make sure that you have the receptionists on board giving out your consent forms and perhaps negotiate slightly longer consultations, or some catch-up slots, to stop you running too far behind.

I used to record my consultations and watch myself and share it with my trainer to critique and with others.

Gloria

- Form a CSA practice group, but ensure that it has a mixture of individuals from different backgrounds. Sometimes there is a tendency for OMGs to form groups among themselves, but this may lead to negative behaviours being reinforced. Ideally you need a group of individuals, both male and female, and from different cultural backgrounds, whom you trust enough to give you honest feedback as to how you are consulting.

ACTION POINT 6

Don't wait to be asked but be proactive and ask some of your colleagues on the day release course to form a practice group with you. If they are not your natural friendship group they may not have thought of practising with you.

Unfortunately when I prepared for the exam I had a group of IMGs without any local graduates. It made it more difficult to understand how local people think and express their feelings.

Shahida

- Take advantage of any extra communication skills sessions that your deanery provides specifically for OMGs. One of the downsides of practising with your English colleagues can be a sense of disillusionment as you realise that your development needs are greater than theirs. Going to sessions with fellow OMGs that have outside facilitation can help to build camaraderie without the likelihood of reinforcing negative behaviours.

ACTION POINT 7

Find out what your deanery offers. If the answer is nothing, then put forward a business case for this to change; after all, some facilitation costs are nothing compared with the cost of an extension to GP training. Even if you don't achieve anything, this will be a good way to improve your negotiation skills for the future.

I gained a lot on the Tuesday sessions when we would have role plays. Learning and watching each other was so valuable. I picked up good things from my colleagues as they were able to correct me and the trainers were also there to teach and support.

Gloria

I have been well supported by the deanery. I have been introduced to the career development unit to improve my linguistic skills. I attend the monthly IMG learning set for CSA preparation.

Rakesh

- Give your trainer, and any colleagues with whom you practice, permission to be honest with you. Sometimes people are afraid to criticise and instead concentrate on building up your confidence, particularly if you have previously failed the exam. While positive feedback is great, what you actually need are constructive suggestions as to how to improve. Make sure that you agree some ground rules within the group as to how you are going to give feedback to one another. This will make sure that you get the maximum educational benefit out of the experience.

ACTION POINT 8

Aim to go away from each debrief or practice session with an action plan of a few areas (no more than three) to work on. Ensure that next time you use the opportunity to review how you have improved in these key areas.

For me I found having a British trainer is more beneficial, because it is their culture and they are able to impart a lot to the trainee, which most IMG trainers don't have. (Although there are some very good IMG trainers.) My trainer had been a GP in England for a long time and he understood what I needed to do.

Anjula

- Practise your explanations of conditions with non-medical friends or family members. This will really develop your skills at phrasing things in patient-friendly language and avoiding jargon. If you just practise with fellow medics then there will inevitably be a tendency for them to say something makes sense when it would not do so to anyone without a medical background. They may not do this deliberately, but once you become used to med-speak it becomes quite difficult to recognise what it is reasonable to expect a non-medic to understand.

ACTION POINT 9

- Check out the Wessex Faculty RCGP CSA case cards (available from the RCGP bookshop) for suggestions of explanations to practise.
- Or what about these YouTube videos from Pennine GP Training: www.pennine-gp-training.co.uk/csa-videos-common-medical-conditions-explained.htm

---

- **Practise your listening skills.** This is the basis of good consulting so use every opportunity, both at work and at home, to develop your active listening skills. If you have children see how well you can encourage them to tell you more about their day; what strategies worked and what had them rushing off to do their homework? Are you listening in order to understand them or in order to be able to reply?

ACTION POINT 10

Try recording an interesting short programme on the radio, or listen to a podcast. Then write a summary of the main points that you heard. Listen to the recording again – how does your written summary compare with what you actually hear?

- Time how long it is before you interrupt a patient in a consultation. Gradually see if you can extend this to a minute – 'the golden minute' – by enhancing your active listening skills.

ACTION POINT 11

In your next surgery, actually time how long it takes until you interrupt a patient. Make a note as to whether your interruption was helpful in moving the consultation on or not.

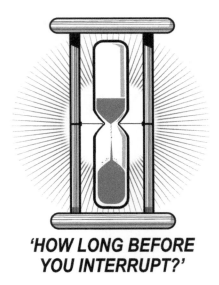

'HOW LONG BEFORE YOU INTERRUPT?'

- Notice when a patient says something you don't understand. Don't then assume that you know what he or she meant (nothing is more able to make an ass of you and me (ass-u-me)!). Instead, experiment with different ways of getting the patient to explain what he or she meant. Don't be afraid that getting the patient to repeat or rephrase something will mean that he or she will lose confidence in you. This is far more likely to happen if, instead of asking, you make an incorrect assumption and so for the rest of the consultation you and the patient are at cross-purposes with each other.

ACTION POINT 12

Make a note of all the phrases that you didn't understand. Then look them up in a dictionary or on your smartphone. Ask a native English speaker if he or she knows what the phrases mean – you may be surprised at how often the native English speaker doesn't know!

- **Notice when patients do not understand what you mean.** Is there a recurring theme? Are you using too much jargon? Are there particular words that you have difficulty pronouncing? Do you speak too fast? Learning to speak more slowly can be a real challenge, but sometimes simply pausing between sentences can have a similar effect and make it much easier for patients to understand you. Also, make sure that patients can hear you. Sometimes OMGs have a tendency to be quite softly spoken and this can be a real challenge for patients. Within the context of the CSA it is a challenge for both role players and examiners! If this is you then you might like to start off speaking slightly louder than usual, as then you will still be able to mirror patients who are speaking softly, such as those who are depressed, by lowering the volume and yet still be able to be heard.

ACTION POINT 13

Make some audio recordings of your consultations (smartphones are great for this). Practise the words that you stumble over or try to think of alternative ways of expressing yourself.

- Think about common scenarios that might come up in the CSA and practise strategies for addressing these. That way you will have a basic structure that you can rely on when it comes to your actual exam. Examples might be breaking bad news or defusing an angry patient.

ACTION POINT 14

Discuss with your colleagues how they might approach these types of consultations. Do they have any constructs that you would find helpful?

● Practise incorporating psychosocial questions into your everyday consultations, rather than just adding them as an afterthought. Being curious about patients as individuals, seeing them as people rather than simply patients, can really help to make your consulting more fluent. A good doctor tends to be a nosy one!

ACTION POINT 15

For each consultation over the next week, make a note of how much non-medical information you have found out about your patients. Are they married? Do they have a family? What does their job actually entail? How has their presenting problem affected their everyday life?

● **Utilise the feedback statements[14] as a guide to help you improve.** You will only be given a feedback statement if two or more examiners have allocated it to you. They are designed as formative tools to help you improve and may be given to both passing and failing candidates. They are linked to the three domains: (1) data gathering, technical and assessment skills, (2) clinical management and (3) interpersonal skills, as well as some global statements. Recognising which domain your feedback comes from can also help you. For example, if you are always marked down on clinical management it may be that it is not so much your communication skills that need improving but rather your knowledge base.

ACTION POINT 16

Look at the RCGP website where there are guides as to how to use the feedback suggestions effectively. These are full of constructive ideas as to what areas you may need to concentrate on for the future.

WORKPLACE-BASED ASSESSMENT

The WPBA component of the MRCGP exam is sometimes underestimated in importance when trainees are concentrating on the exam components of AKT and CSA. It also has a difficult role to play in that it is a combination of both a formative learning tool and a summative assessment of your progress and eventual competence within the workplace. It is certainly possible to pass both the exam components of MRCGP and yet still fail on the WPBA aspect. Indeed, almost 50% of the trainees in our deanery who required extensions to their training last year did so for failure to progress with WPBA. However, it is unlikely to be what you write in your e-portfolio that causes problems; rather, it is more likely to be the absence of evidence that is the issue.

There is no doubt that the e-portfolio is more suited to naturally reflective individuals who find words an effective learning medium. It is much harder for those who prefer a visual or auditory form of learning to demonstrate their learning effectively through the tool available. However, it is a tool that is here to stay and so you need to be able to use it effectively. It also bears significant similarities to what will be expected of you once you are qualified to demonstrate your commitment to continuing your professional development and preparing for revalidation.

So it makes sense to try to maximise the use of the e-portfolio as a formative learning tool, as this will make it much less onerous to complete. It will also probably mean that you easily pass the summative elements of this component.

> I find the portfolio difficult because of the language. But it does mean that I can show my learning from patients, and I like that. It is better to use it regularly than to panic at the last minute. Sometimes we forget it because we are stressed about the exams but that is not right. It can help you.
>
> Maria

THE FORMAL WORKPLACE-BASED ASSESSMENT TOOLS

WPBA is a mixture of formal assessment tools and a formative learning log. We will come to the learning log later, but first let's look at the more formal components (*see* next page).

Case-based discussion (CbD)	This is a structured interview designed to test your professional judgement in a clinical situation. Your responsibility is to provide your assessor (who may be your ES or CS) with the clinical records of two cases (at St1 or St2) or four cases (at St3) for them to choose a case from. The cases should not be ones that you have previously discussed in a debriefing session and they should reflect the scope of your clinical practice. Particularly at St3 you might like to take into account those areas of the curriculum, or professional competences, for which you have less evidence.
Clinical Evaluation Exercise (Mini-CEX) (the hospital equivalent of a COT – *see* following entry)	This provides a snapshot of how you interact with patients in a secondary care setting, looking at your clinical skills, attitudes and behaviours. Your responsibility is to identify clinical encounters that might form the basis of a mini-CEX, and also to reflect on the feedback that you are given within your learning log. Getting different individuals to observe you at different times can be really useful. The observer could be a staff grade doctor, nurse practitioner, clinical nurse specialist, an experienced specialty registrar (St4 or above) or consultant. The observer should not be a peer – a fellow GP trainee or specialty trainee at a similar stage in training, or more junior.
Consultation observation tool (COT)	This tool gives your ES (or CS) the chance to make some holistic judgements about your consulting ability. It can be based either on direct observation of your consulting, such as in a joint surgery, or on reviewing videoed consultations. Your responsibility is to ensure that you have some suitable video recordings (not more than 15 minutes' duration), with appropriate patient consent for your ES, or CS, to review. Alternatively, ensure that you have some joint surgeries scheduled. Ideally a mixture of video analysis and joint surgeries will be most useful. The cases need to reflect the breadth of your clinical workload and include at least one child (under 10 years of age), one older adult (over 75 years of age) and one demonstrating mental health problems.
Direct Observation of Procedural Skills (DOPS)	This is designed to check your ability to undertake important and technically challenging procedures. There are eight mandatory DOPS that you need to complete during your GP training: 1. application of a simple dressing 2. breast examination 3. cervical cytology 4. female genital examination 5. male genital examination 6. prostate examination 7. rectal examination 8. testing for blood glucose.

Direct Observation of Procedural Skills (DOPS)	Your responsibility is to ensure that you get someone appropriate to observe you undertaking these. These would include those who can observe a mini-CEX (*see* previous entry). Your DOPS can be undertaken at any point in your GP training, but your ES needs to be confident of your ability to undertake them in a primary care setting. This means that it is possible, although unusual, that your ES will ask you to repeat some of the DOPS that you got signed up early in the hospital components of your training. Assessments undertaken during your Foundation programme cannot be carried over.
	There are also 11 optional DOPS that you can get signed up (look at www.rcgp.org. uk).
Multi source feedback (MSF)	This is used to collect the opinion of your colleagues on your clinical performance and professional behaviour. This is good preparation for revalidation as MSF is a cornerstone of this also.
	Your responsibility is to identify five to ten individuals (minimum), depending on whether you are in primary or secondary care, who would be willing and able to provide feedback on your abilities. You should also reflect upon their suggestions for your development so as to be able to demonstrate change between the two rounds of feedback.
Clinical supervisor's report (CSR)	While in secondary care, your ES will not have an opportunity to observe your clinical work and interaction with patients on a regular basis. So this report gives the consultant with whom you work regularly an opportunity to give feedback as to how you are doing, as well as possible areas for development.
	Your responsibility is to identify (with the aid of your GP team if necessary) the person who would be best placed to provide this feedback and get him or her to complete a CSR. You can maximise the potential of this by also trying to meet with your CS early in the post, so as to identify particular competences that you would like to develop within the post that are particularly relevant to general practice.
	You need a CSR for *each* clinical post, so if your posts are 3 months' duration then you will need two CSRs for each 6-month review.
	When in primary care, whether you need a CSR depends on whether your GP trainer who is acting as your CS is also your ES. If he or she is both your ES and your CS then it is not compulsory to undertake a CSR, but they are still sometimes done as they can provide added value.
Patient Satisfaction Questionnaire (PSQ)	This tool provides feedback on your communication skills from patients, particularly your ability to gain rapport and demonstrate empathy and relationship building. Again it is a cornerstone of revalidation for the future.
	Your responsibility is to ensure that you get the practice on board at the appropriate time, such that you manage to get 40 fully completed questionnaires from patients.
	There is a strict timescale over which to submit these so it is worth reading these carefully before starting the process. You may also want to give out more than 40 questionnaires as it is likely that at least one or two will not be fully completed and so won't count, which could leave you short.
	You will also need to have identified someone, often a practice manager, who would be prepared to enter these onto your e-portfolio.

THE FORMAL COMPONENTS OF WORKPLACE-BASED ASSESSMENT: WHAT HAPPENS WHEN?

Keeping on top of the formal components of WPBA is the first step in making the most use of it, developmentally as well as in a summative way. For if you are trying to cram in several mini-CEXs or CbDs just before your educational review then you will inevitably be focusing just on getting them completed rather than on their usefulness.

The following tables clearly lay out the minimum requirements in order to progress with WPBA.

GP specialty training year 1	
Minimum requirements before 6-month review	3 × COT (if in primary care) or 3 × mini-CEX (if in secondary care)
	3 × CbD
	1 × MSF (five clinicians if in secondary care plus five non-clinicians if in primary care)
	DOPS, as appropriate
	CSR (one for each job)
Minimum requirements prior to 12-month review (the deadline for which may well actually be 11 months)	3 × COT (if in primary care) or 3 × mini-CEX (if in secondary care)
	3 × CbD
	1 × MSF (five clinicians if in secondary care plus five non-clinicians if in primary care)
	1 × PSQ (if in primary care)
	DOPS, as appropriate
	CSR (one for each job)

GP specialty training year 2	
Minimum requirements before 18-month review	3 × COT (if in primary care) or 3 × mini-CEX (if in secondary care)
	3 × CbD
	1 × PSQ (if in primary care and not already completed in St1)
	DOPS, as appropriate
	CSR (one for each job)
Minimum requirements prior to 24-month review (the deadline for which may well actually be 23 months)	3 × COT (if in primary care) or 3 × mini-CEX (if in secondary care)
	3 × CbD
	1 × PSQ (if in primary care and not already completed in St1 or earlier in St2)
	DOPS, as appropriate
	CSR (one for each job)

GP specialty training year 3 (if whole year is in primary care)	
Minimum requirements prior to 30-month review	6 × COT
	6 × CbD
	1 × MSF (five clinicians and five non-clinicians)
	DOPS, as appropriate
Minimum requirements prior to the final review (the deadline for which may well actually be 34 months)	6 × COT
	6 × CbD
	1 × MSF (five clinicians and five non-clinicians)
	1 × PSQ
	DOPS, as appropriate

If you are in an innovative training post, or working on a less than full-time basis then it is probably best to check out the requirements online (www.rcgp.org.uk).

The *minimum* numbers of each assessment are clearly displayed on your e-portfolio and (assuming you are full-time) these numbers will turn from red to green once you have the requisite number. These numbers will reset with each ES review so you cannot 'carry over' any extra assessments from one review to another. This only serves to emphasise the need to arrange these reviews on a timely basis or you will find yourself cramming in assessments in order to meet the deadlines.

You should remember, however, that these numbers are the *minimum* numbers that are required. By the end of your training you will need to be able to provide evidence that you are competent for licensing across *all* the professional competences. These formal assessments can form a useful source of such evidence alongside the learning log. This may mean that you end up completing more than the minimum numbers in order to get sufficient breadth of coverage, as each assessment is unlikely to cover all the competences. If done well, the formal assessments can also be really useful as a formative exercise, identifying areas of possible development for the future. This is particularly true for those done in a primary care setting, with enthusiastic, well-informed ESs.

ACTION POINT 17

Review your e-portfolio. Are you on track to complete the necessary assessments? Make a plan as to how to get one of the formal assessments – such as a CbD, mini-CEX, COT – done in the next 2 weeks.

THE LEARNING LOG

Alongside the formal assessments of WPBA sits the learning log. This is the record of your learning, both from patients in the form of clinical encounters and also from your formal educational activities such as tutorials, reading and e-learning. If you put in entries on a regular basis, such as two to three clinical encounters a week, you will soon have a rich source of evidence of your learning, and also be able to identify potential areas of weakness or learning need. It is the quality of the entries that is of primary importance but clearly there is also a minimum level of quantity in order to enable judgements to be made. Most deaneries would expect a minimum of 100 learning log entries each year.

TYPES OF LEARNING LOG ENTRY

Sometimes people struggle to know what sort of entries they should make under each of the possible types of log entry. To be honest, so long as the information is there, and can be found by your ES and ARCP panel, it is not too important. However, here is a quick guide to what goes where.

Clinical encounters	PUNs and DENs, case analyses, case reviews, any external clinical sessions attended (e.g. outpatient clinics)
Professional conversations	ES meetings, feedback/appraisal on day-to-day basis, discussions on health-related topics or related to attitudes, skills or organisational management
Placement planning meeting	Record of initial meetings with your CS or ES detailing your aims for your next placement
Tutorials	Half-day release, tutorials in practice, consultation skills tutorials, tutorials on non-clinical stuff (i.e. IT training)
Audits or projects	Audit, any work linked to the QOF, quality improvement work
Significant event analysis	Reflection on significant event (which may be negative or positive)
e-learning modules	Record e-learning sessions (good ones – BMJ Learning, RCGP eGP updates, GPnotebook GEMs (GPnotebook educational modules) and Doctors.net)
Reading	Books, papers, protocols, articles on web, films, plays, and so forth
Courses or certificates	Life support courses, deanery-led courses (e.g. child health surveillance, mock CSA courses), external courses
Lectures and seminars	Protected learning time events (e.g. in-house education, lectures in hospital setting, seminars)
Academic activity	Used primarily by academic clinical fellows to record research and academic courses – this is to enable it to be easily identifiable by the academic supervisor (who is often neither the ES nor the CS)
OOH sessions	Document all sessions (note not extended hours), including the duration of the session in the first line of the entry, and also attach the session sheet to the log entry

At the moment there are no nationally agreed prerequisites of the type of entry needed for your learning log, with the exception of OOH and resuscitation status (*see* 'The Extra Bits!' *section* later in this chapter). However, some deaneries have made local recommendations regarding naturally occurring evidence, such as significant event analysis (SEA) and audit, so it makes sense to check with your local deanery. It is possible to challenge locally led requirements but it is probably easier just to try to make sure that you complete them if at all possible. Also, given that WPBA can be seen as good preparation for annual appraisal and revalidation as a qualified GP, recording SEAs (which do form part of the mandatory requirements for this) would be good practice. Most GPStRs would easily find two SEAs, particularly if you include positive events, to reflect upon during each year of their GP training.

WHAT MAKES A GOOD LEARNING LOG ENTRY?

A good entry will include evidence that you have been able to reflect on your practice and use concrete experience to try out new ideas and then observe what happens when you implement them. This relates back to the learning cycle that we explored in Chapter 2: Learning How to Learn. It includes *what* (i.e. what actually happened), then *so what* (this is the reflecting part of the entry, thinking about why does that matter) and *now what* (moving on to the next stage).

The *so what* and *now what* aspects of the log are the most interesting parts and also the areas that demonstrate to the reader that you have learnt from the encounter. So it makes sense for those to be the areas of the log entry that you spend most time on. This means that good learning log entries are often shaped like a Christmas tree, or are bottom heavy. Some people find it helpful to try completing the bottom boxes first, as we are all usually more enthusiastic when we start, and it also means that the entry is often less repetitive. Otherwise the danger is that you actually end up spending loads of time describing what happened and then lose your motivation before thinking about the learning points, or end up mixing together the learning and the description.

It is also helpful to think about your learning in the *so what* and *now what* aspects in relation to general practice and how you might approach a similar situation in primary care. For example, if you were involved in a resuscitation scenario in secondary care this might prompt you to consider how GPs maintain their resuscitation skills and what equipment and drugs might be available to you if a cardiac arrest occurred in a GP surgery. Or if you came across a child with complex developmental issues, then, rather than concentrating on the fine details of an obscure genetic condition, you might like to reflect on the services and support available to patients with disabilities, and their carers, in the community. Or even the common, more generic issue as to how GPs deal with patients with rare conditions that they are unfamiliar with, as this will definitely be something that you come across again during your career.

ACTION POINT 18

For your next learning log entry, try completing the bottom boxes first, then moving on to the top boxes where you describe what happened. Does this alter the shape of your entry?

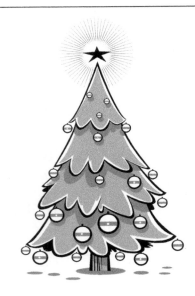

When writing a log entry it also makes sense to remember that it is a professional document that others will read, so think about the language that you use. Try not to be judgemental of patients or colleagues, although of course you should feel able to make constructive criticism when it is justified. Remember also to retain confidentiality, removing identifiable patient details. If you want to be able to refer back to the patient to see what happened subsequently, then you could include his or her EMIS number (or similar), as this will uniquely identify the patient for you, without making him or her identifiable to the reader. Make sure that you not only include the factual elements but also that you think about how something made you feel, for it is often our emotions that lead us to change rather than our intellect. Remember to spellcheck the document, or at the very least to read it through before releasing it, as once your ES has read your shared log entry you will no longer be able to edit it, although if you remember something later, or there are relevant subsequent events, you can add these as a comment. Some people find it easier to write their entries in a Word document and then copy and paste them into the e-portfolio. It is up to you whether you take that approach, but remember that if you are writing directly into the e-portfolio you must make sure that you save it regularly, as the security features will lock you out after only 5–10 minutes and you would not want to lose all your hard work!

Remember, entries do not need to be perfect. They are of most value when shared soon after the learning event occurred. This means that any input from your ES can actually influence future events. Some trainees store up entries for months on end and then release them in batches to their ES. This is not really fair on your ES and will significantly affect the use of the e-portfolio as a formative educational tool. It is also likely to raise concerns about your progress from your wider educational team, as they will probably be regularly reviewing your learning log to look at the number of entries that you are entering, if not the quality of their detail.

EXAMPLES OF A LEARNING LOG ENTRY

Sometimes it is easier to put ideas into practice if you can see an example! The following two learning log entries are based on the same clinical scenario, which actually occurred during one of my (MF) recent surgeries.

The first entry is written as we might expect an St1 to complete a log entry, whereas the second entry is that of an St3.

GPSt1 in practice

What happened?

It was a Wednesday morning surgery and mum came in with her 9-month-old baby. She told me that over the past 2 weeks the child had been reluctant to lie flat, and started crying and drawing her legs up when she was put down. She was still feeding OK and was fine in between times, so mum just thought she had colic, particularly as she was having loose nappies. Over the past 2 days, however, her nappies had changed colour to a burgundy colour, which mum thought was unusual, so she had brought her to see if this was of any significance.

I vaguely remembered that 'redcurrant jelly stools' was a clinical feature of intussusception so I quickly looked this up in the *Ox Handbook of GP* and the child was the right age. I then examined the child but there was nothing to find and the child appeared to be completely well. However, I thought I should get the child assessed to rule out intussusception so I referred the child into paediatrics.

What, if anything, happened subsequently?

Child was seen by the paediatrics department and a barium enema was performed, which served to both confirm the diagnosis and to treat the condition.

What did you learn? What will you do differently in future?

Even apparently healthy children can be hiding a significant underlying medical condition and it is important to take a clear history and respond to the parents' concerns. Also, if you are not sure of something it is better to look it up, or ask someone, rather than just ignoring the sense that something is important, if only you could remember it!

What further learning needs did you identify?

- How to assess a sick child, so as to better able to discuss the situation with the paediatrics department.
- Clinical presentations of common and important paediatric emergencies.

How and when will you address these?

- Read the relevant chapters of the *Ox Handbook of GP*.
- Arrange tutorial on paediatrics with my trainer.

GPSt3 in practice

What happened?

A mum brought in her 9-month-old baby who for the past 2 weeks had been reluctant to lie flat, and started crying and drawing her legs up when she was put down. In between times she was completely healthy but over the past 2 days her stools had become burgundy coloured and mum wondered if that was significant. I remembered that this could be a presenting sign of intussusception so I phoned the paediatric registrar even though clinical examination of the child was unremarkable. The paediatric registrar asked me what the child's blood pressure was and I explained that I had not done it, although I did have the heart rate and cap refill time (which were normal). I felt that the paediatric registrar was being obstructive but I found it difficult to express my concerns about her response, as mum was listening to my part of the conversation. Before making the call I had explained to mum that I thought this could represent a serious underlying problem that we needed to rule out and that she would need to go to the local district general hospital, which is 20 miles away. Mum had difficulty taking this on board (as the child seemed so healthy), so it was even more awkward that I felt I was having to 'persuade' the paediatrics registrar.

What, if anything, happened subsequently?

Eventually the paediatrics registrar accepted the case, as I think she realised I was not going to back down. So the child was seen by the paediatrics department and a barium enema was performed, which served to both confirm the diagnosis and to treat the condition. I learnt this from mum (am still awaiting the discharge summary), who wrote me a thank-you note for my care and concern.

What did you learn? What will you do differently in future?

I learnt not to ignore my gut instincts,* even if someone else who is more senior than me is challenging it, and also to stand up for my clinical acumen, as it is obviously inappropriate to measure blood pressure in a 9-month-old in general practice. I knew that if I had not sent the child in, I would have continued to worry about her. I need to think about whether or not I make telephone referrals in front of the patient when I know they have the potential to be difficult.

What further learning needs did you identify?

How do other GPs make their emergency referrals? Is it better to discuss your thoughts with the patient before or after discussing with secondary care?

How and when will you address these?

- Discuss with my trainer and also with the other St3s on the day release course.

Hopefully these two examples demonstrate how your thinking could move on from St1 to St3. Initially the learner focused on the clinical aspects of the situation, whereas the more experienced learner thinks beyond this to the more challenging aspects of liaising with colleagues and trusting your gut instincts.

Both entries include a reasonable amount of descriptive material, as this is important to be able to set the context in this particular situation. However, this is not at the expense of thinking about the learning opportunities that the case presented and also helps to make it an interesting entry for the ES to read. Neither of the entries are particularly lengthy and there is no emphasis on the writing quality, beyond checking the spelling and ensuring that it makes sense to the reader. Some entries will not need as much description to be able to put the entry into context.

ACTION POINT 19

Thinking of the two learning log entry examples provided, think about what curriculum statement headings it might be appropriate to link them to.

Phrase notes
* 'gut instincts' – following your intuition

WHAT CAN I EXPECT OF MY EDUCATIONAL SUPERVISOR?

Your ES will be a key person in helping you to progress through your GP training so it makes sense to invest in this relationship early on. You are likely to have one ES for the entire duration of your GP training. However, in some areas you will change ES partway through so as to ensure that your GP trainer, when in a GP practice, is always also your ES. In most areas the ES is a GP trainer although in some deaneries the GP training PDs take on this role. If this is the case in your deanery then it is worth remembering that each PD is probably fulfilling this role for multiple individuals.

You should arrange to meet your ES soon after starting your GP training so as to get to know each other. One of his or her key roles can be in helping you to identify the learning opportunities in your hospital jobs so as to maximise the educational value of these posts. Also, getting to know your ES means that you will be more able to confide in him or her should difficulties arise, either within your jobs or in your life outside, which then affects your training. It is also possible that your ES may well invite you to practice-based social events that will make you feel part of the practice team and help facilitate your time in general practice, as well as give you valuable opportunities to practise your English and find out more about British culture.

Apart from this pastoral aspect, one of the main roles of your ES is in commenting on your learning log and undertaking formal educational reviews with you on a 6-monthly basis. If you are in practice with your ES, he or she may also be involved in some of the formal assessments of WPBA, such as CbDs and COTs.

A good ES will read and comment on your learning log regularly, although you probably cannot expect him or her to comment on every entry. If it appears that your ES is not reading and/or commenting regularly, then feel free to take this up with your PD, as this is one of his or her training responsibilities. If you release your entries regularly and soon after the event occurred, then the comments from your ES may well identify future learning for you, or even influence your future management of the patient. Often this will take the form of questioning, in a Socratic style.

> Having a good ES is important. My ES made comments on my entries that made me think differently. This really helped me to understand. It also made me feel it was worth spending time on my log.
>
> Yomi

If we go back to the learning log entry examples regarding the child with intussusception, then examples of the comments of a good ES might be as follows.

> *ES comments (for GPSt1)*: What an interesting and unusual case to reflect on. How did you assess whether the child was healthy? Are you familiar with the NICE traffic light system

for assessing sick children? How did you explain your actions to mum if she was not particularly worried about the child? What other resources could you use within a consultation, to refresh your knowledge and/or give to patients?

ES comments (for GPSt3): Have you reached any conclusions as to whether or not to make future phone calls in front of the patient? What about referral letters – could you dictate them with the patient in the room? What have you done with the thank-you letter? Have you been in touch with the family since? This case would form the basis of an interesting CbD if you would like to take it further.

In both instances the ES has managed to take the particular example given by the GPStR and extend that to be applicable to other situations that he or she might come across in the future within general practice. So with the aid of a good ES even the more obscure clinical encounters can become much more relevant. They have also managed to suggest how to utilise one of the formal assessment tools in a meaningful way rather than just as a tick-box exercise.

The other way in which your ES interacts with your learning log is by validating your linkage with the curriculum headings that you have identified. The ES will also validate your entry against the professional competencies. By adding professional competencies your ES is not saying that you have achieved competence in that area but, rather, that you have provided evidence of learning and development in that particular area. Some ESs find it helpful, particularly later in your training when you are trying to fill any potential gaps in your evidence, if you can target your learning log entries toward a particular professional competency and signpost this clearly to them.

There are 12 professional competencies that you need to demonstrate competence in by the end of your GP training.
1. **Communication and consultation skills**: this is about how you communicate with patients and your use of recognised consultation techniques.
2. **Practising holistically**: this is about your ability to operate in physical, psychological, socio-economic and cultural dimensions, taking into account feelings as well as thoughts.
3. **Data gathering and interpretation**: this is about how you gather and use data for clinical judgement, your choice of examination and investigations and their interpretation.
4. **Making a diagnosis and making decisions**: this is about you demonstrating a conscious, structured approach to how you make decisions.
5. **Clinical management**: this is about your ability to manage common clinical medical conditions in primary care.
6. **Managing medical complexity**: this is about the aspects of care beyond managing straightforward problems, including the management of co-morbidity, uncertainty and risk, and the approach to health rather than just illness.

7. **Primary care administration and information management and technology**: this is about the appropriate use of primary care administration systems, effective record keeping and information technology for the benefit of patient care.
8. **Working with colleagues and in teams**: this is about how you work effectively with other professionals to ensure good patient care, including the sharing of information with colleagues.
9. **Community orientation**: this is about the management of the health and social care of the practice population and local community.
10. **Maintaining performance, learning and teaching**: this is about how you maintain both your own performance and effective CPD and that of others.
11. **Maintaining an ethical approach to practice**: this is about how you communicate with patients, and your use of recognised consultation techniques.
12. **Fitness to practise**: this is about your awareness of when your own performance, conduct or health, or that of others might put patients at risk and what action you take to protect patients.

You will find more details of these on the RCGP website or in *The Condensed Curriculum Guide*.[3]

The personal development plan

The PDP is the final cornerstone of WPBA and is unfortunately often neglected. Used properly it can be an incredibly useful tool and will also put you in a good position for thinking about your CPD once you are working in independent practice. Formulating and maintaining your PDP is a key part of annual appraisal, and subsequently revalidation.

The idea of a PDP is that it is a way of recording your learning needs to fulfil areas of potential weakness as well as those that are more aspirational, and seek to extend your current scope of practice. The emphasis should be on your *personal*, professional development, what *you*, as an individual need or want to achieve over the coming period. This means that including essential achievements that are applicable to *all* GP trainees, such as passing your CSA, is not maximising the potential of a good PDP. You will find more information on this subject in Chapter 2: Learning How to Learn.

You will be able to identify some areas for your PDP from your learning log entries, but these tend to be about potential areas of weakness rather than those that seek to enhance your practice. The important thing to remember is that your PDP should be a living document that you need to revisit regularly. It is not enough to simply export a learning log entry to your PDP. You also need to think about *how* you will fulfil that particular learning need and then record once you have completed it.

ACTION POINT 20

Look at your PDP with a critical eye:

- Have you made any recent entries?
- Is there a balance between addressing areas of potential weakness and being aspirational?
- Have you completed any of your PDP entries? Have you recorded this?

THE EXTRA BITS!

By the time you get to the end of your training there are also a few other mandatory requirements before you can get signed up for your CCT. It is worth mentioning these to make sure that you don't get caught out at the last minute!

The first thing that you will need to have signed off is completion of your OOH training. Assuming that you have spent 18 months of a 3-year training programme in a primary care setting, you will need to undertake a minimum of 107 hours of OOH experience, which roughly equates to 1 × 6-hour shift for every month in a primary care setting. Extended hours and practice duty days do not count toward this total. In some areas there is a real pressure on places for GPStRs to undertake OOH sessions, so you need to get this organised on a regular basis, rather than hoping for the best at the last minute!

> I wish I had sorted out my OOHs earlier. Instead I found myself cramming in sessions at the last minute when I would have been better practising for my CSA.
>
> Daniel

Second, your ES will have to sign you up as competent in basic life support (BLS) and automated external defibrillation use. Most practices have a regular programme of resuscitation training, but this does not always incorporate the role of automated external defibrillators, so you may need to make sure that this is covered, or find an alternative source of updating. If you hold a valid ALS certificate that you undertook during your GP training (but not as part of a Foundation programme), then this will count as an alternative. You need to make sure that you upload the actual certificate to your e-portfolio as proof that you have successfully completed this training.

The final piece of mandatory training that you may need to include is evidence that you have completed some child protection training. Completing the professional competencies of WPBA will mean that you gain the equivalence of Level 3 certification in safeguarding. However, many practice and OOH providers will require you to provide proof, by means of a certificate, that you have undertaken Level 3 training in safeguarding children and vulnerable adults. You will also probably be expected to supply such a certificate to future practices if you are exploring locum work once you are qualified. As with BLS, this training may be done within the practice but not always (as it tends to be on a 3-year cycle), so you need to explore how else you might achieve this. In some areas it features as part of the day release training programme, but obviously you would need to make sure that you are not on annual leave that day!

ACTION POINT 21

Find out when the day release course or practice is going to cover BLS and safeguarding issues. If there are no suitable dates scheduled, then make a plan as to how you will address these learning needs.

Hopefully this chapter has given you some suggestions as to how to maximise your chances of success at the MRCGP exam. The RCGP website also has a lot of useful information that is worth exploring and you can also contact the exams department for advice if, for example, you are concerned about reasonable adjustments being made for a disability. Inevitably, the statistics suggest that some of you will have difficulty with the assessments. Keeping a positive outlook is essential, as well as keeping things in perspective. You will have faced other challenges in your life, some far more extreme than this, and you have come through them.

So think positive, work hard and do not be too proud to take all the help that is on offer to you.

REFERENCES

1. Royal College of General Practitioners (RCGP). *Being a General Practitioner*. London: RCGP; 2013. Available at: www.rcgp.org.uk/gp-training-and-exams/~/media/Files/GP-training-and-exams/Curriculum-2012/RCGP-Curriculum-1-Being-a-GP.ashx (accessed 9 September 2013).
2. Royal College of General Practitioners (RCGP). *The GP Curriculum: overview*. London: RCGP; 2013. Available at: www.rcgp.org.uk/gp-training-and-exams/gp-curriculum-overview.aspx (accessed 9 September 2013).
3. Riley B, Haynes J, Field S. *The Condensed Curriculum Guide*. 2nd ed. London: Royal College of General Practitioners; 2012.
4. Miller GE. The assessment of clinical skills/performance. *Acad Med*. 1990: 65(9 Suppl.): S63–7.
5. Royal College of General Practitioners (RCGP). *The Applied Knowledge Test Content Guide*. London: RCGP; 2013. Available at: www.rcgp.org.uk/gp-training-and-exams/mrcgp-exam-overview/~/media/Files/GP-training-and-exams/AKT%20page/Content%20Guide%20August%202013.ashx (accessed 9 September 2013).
6. Esmail A, Roberts C. *Independent Review of the Membership of the Royal College of General Practitioners (MRCGP) Examination*. Manchester: University of Manchester;

2013. Available at: www.gmc-uk.org/MRCGP_Final_Report__18th_September_2013.pdf_53516840.pdf (accessed 23 October 2013).

7. Royal College of General Practitioners (RCGP). *MRCGP Statistics: 2010–11 Report 2010–2011*. London: RCGP; 2011. Available at: www.rcgp.org.uk/gp-training-and-exams/mrcgp-exam-overview/~/media/Files/GP-training-and-exams/Annual%20reports/MRCGP%20Statistics%20201011%20draft%20at%20071111.ashx (accessed 13 March 2014).

8. Wakeford R. International medical graduates' relative under-performance in the MRCGP AKT and CSA examinations. *Educ Prim Care.* 2012; **23**(3): 148–52.

9. Patterson F, Denney ML, Wakeford R, *et al.* Fair and equal assessment in postgraduate training? A future research agenda. *Br J Gen Pract.* 2011; **61**(593): 712–13.

10. Denney ML, Freeman A, Wakeford R. MRCGP CSA: are the examiners biased, favouring their own by sex, ethnicity, and degree source? *Br J Gen Pract.* 2013; **63**(616): e718–25.

11. General Medical Council (GMC). *Annual Specialty Reports of Exam Success: report year 2010/11*. London: GMC; 2012.

12. Royal College of General Practitioners/COPMED. *Dress Codes for Postgraduate GP Recruitment, Training and Assessment.* Available at: www.rcgp.org.uk/gp-training-and-exams/mrcgp-exam-overview/~/media/Files/GP-training-and-exams/Dress-codes-for-postgraduate-GP-recruitment-training-and-assessment.ashx (accessed 9 September 2013).

13. General Medical Council (GMC). *Good Medical Practice (2013)*. London: GMC: 2013. Available at: www.gmc-uk.org/guidance/good_medical_practice.asp (accessed 9 September 2013).

14. Royal College of General Practitioners (RCGP). *MRCGP Clinical Skills Assessment CSA Candidate Feedback.* Available at: www.rcgp.org.uk/gp-training-and-exams/mrcgp-exam-overview/~/media/Files/GP-training-and-exams/CSA%20page/Exams%20Guidance%20on%20interpreting%20CSA%20feedback%20v12%20SRKHJACAF%20160114.ashx (accessed 9 September 2013).

CHAPTER 6

What next?

Getting your CCT is just the first part; now you need to think about what sort of GP you want to be.

This chapter aims to explain some of the practicalities involved in getting your next job. However, the first step is thinking about what this dream job would look like. This may well be the first time that you have thought about such things since getting a place on your GP training scheme. So it is worth taking a step back and thinking about what your core values are that would influence such a decision. Some people find that easy to do whereas others find such abstract thinking more difficult. Breaking it down into thinking about what sort of practice you want to work in can help to stimulate this thought process. However, it is sometimes worth stepping back and trying to understand *why* you have reached a particular conclusion. There is no right or wrong answer; the skill is in knowing what is the right answer *for you*, which may look very different from the right answer for one of us or for another of your colleagues. What you conclude will be informed by your personal and family circumstances and your priorities in life, as well as your cultural and religious beliefs.

WHAT SORT OF PRACTICE DO YOU WANT TO WORK IN?

During your GP training you will probably have only had the opportunity to work in two or three different practices at most. It makes sense to have made the most of this by choosing practices with different practice profiles, styles of working and computer systems. You should also take any opportunities that present themselves to undertake a practice swap for a week or two, or even just to visit those of your colleagues from the day release course.

Hopefully this will have given some ideas as to what sort of practice you would most like to work in. Things you might like to consider are listed as follows.

● Is it a rural, semi-rural or urban practice?

- Is it a training or teaching practice?
- Are they dispensing or non-dispensing?
- Is the practice population generally young or old?
- What is the main socio-economic status of the practice population?
- Are there lots of non-native English speakers? If so what is the predominant language used? Could you consult in this language or will you need to use an interpreter? (If English is not your first language either, it may be very exhausting to have to work through an interpreter to a third language.)
- Does the practice population have any special characteristics? For example, is it near a military base? Are there lots of university students? Are there lots of asylum seekers?
- Do they welcome individuals with outside interests?
- What are the practice priorities? Earning potential? Patient care? Work–life balance?
- Does the practice represent a particular viewpoint to the local community? For example, is it the local 'Christian practice?' What does this actually mean?

If you find a practice that you quite like but which has aspects that you are less keen on, such as an old computer system or a clunky appointments system, then you need to ask yourself two questions:

1. How easy would this be to change? Some things, such as the practice ethos, are fundamental to how a practice functions and it would be virtually impossible to change.
2. How important is it for you to be able to get the practice to change? If they were not to change would you still want to work there?

Be realistic about what you can achieve!

ACTION POINT 1

Make a list of the characteristics of your ideal practice. Now decide which of these you consider to be essential and which you consider to be desirable. Remember to think about both positive and negative characteristics – that is, things that would make you want to work somewhere and things that would put you off.

HOW DO YOU SEE YOURSELF BEING EMPLOYED?

Over time general practice within the UK has changed considerably. This has increased the different employment options that will be available to you once you qualify.

Broadly speaking, in terms of a clinical role within general practice, there are now three main options: (1) GP partner (also known as a GP principal), (2) salaried and (3) locum, but these break down into further options. It is worth remembering that different models may suit you at different times in your career and that it is possible to move from one to another, although some are clearly designed with a more long-term perspective in mind. Some day release courses include sessions later in the year, when different people come and share their perspectives, which can be really useful in challenging your ideas.

GP partner (also known as a GP principal)

This is the traditional way in which UK general practice was organised and involves you being a businessman (or businesswoman) as well as a clinician. You will usually buy a share of the business, which will probably involve taking out a business loan. You will then be responsible, with your partners, for the smooth running of the business, including employing all the staff. You will not be paid a salary but you will take 'drawings', which come out of the profit that you make as a business. Drawings are effectively the amount of money that you, as a partnership, decide to pay yourselves each month. Some practices choose to have lower drawings, which then raises the possibility of an end-of-year bonus, whereas others pay themselves more each month but risk having to repay the practice if they do not do as well as they had originally predicted. This means that your earnings have the potential to go down as well as up. Indeed, recently most GP partners have seen their take-home income fall as expenses have increased significantly. However, GP partners do still tend to earn more than their salaried colleagues.

As a partner you will have a voice in the running of the practice, not only from a clinical perspective but also as a business. This would include making decisions about issues such as how many practice nurses to employ or whether to redecorate the waiting room.

Depending upon the practice premises you may also hold equity in the building. Just as with your home, you will make mortgage payments and it is worth remembering that the value of the property can go down as well as up. Occasionally you can become a partner without gaining a share in the property, in which case you will not be involved in decisions that centre on the building.

In the past, people tended to become partners and stay in the same practice for their entire working life. Now it is quite common for people to change practice, even within the same geographical area, although you would probably need to be thinking of at least a 5-year commitment before taking on a partnership (recognising that of course your circumstances might change). So it may not suit you to take on a partnership, at least initially, if you are waiting for your life partner to complete his or her training before deciding where you would like to settle from a geographical perspective.

There are lots of things to consider when thinking of applying for a partnership but here is an outline of some of them.

- What do they consider to be full-time? This may be eight or nine sessions (or very occasionally even ten!) depending on the partnership.
- If you are applying for a less than full-time partnership, are there already any other part-time partners? How will this fit with the timings of any important meetings? If you are to be the first less than full-timer, have they thought through how this will work?
- What is their view of outside interests? How do they treat the income from such activities – is it shared practice income or given to each individual separately? (Often outside interests pay less than your partnership earnings, so establishing what happens to this money can have significant financial implications.)
- Do they own their practice building? Are they all property-owning partners?
- How do they make decisions? Do these have to be unanimous or just a majority?
- How long will it take you to reach parity, when you will be on an equal footing (and take equal pay) with the other partners?
- What is the balance between partners and salaried doctors? How do they treat their salaried employees? How often do their salaried GPs change?
- What is their meeting schedule like? Do they have regular clinical meetings as well as business meetings? What about educational events? Which members of staff come to the meetings?
- What are the demographics of the existing partners? Will you be the only man or woman? Is it likely that they will all retire at the same time?
- How stable is the partnership? If a number of partners have left recently what was the reason for this?
- What sort of list system do they operate? Is it a strictly enforced personal list system (where patients *always* consult with the same doctor), which is great for continuity but has other downsides, or a more flexible 'usual doctor' system?
- What are the relationships like between the partners? Are any of them married to each other? This will obviously affect holidays (assuming they would like to go together) and may also affect decision-making. Think very carefully before agreeing to be the third partner with a married couple.
- How long have the rest of the staff been there? If all the receptionists have been employed for years, then that suggests that they are probably reasonable employers.
- Is their practice list size increasing or decreasing? If it is falling what efforts have they made to try to reverse this trend?

- Do they have any branch surgeries? Are they a dispensing practice (where they effectively also run a pharmacy) for some, or all, of their patients?
- Are they a training practice? What about an undergraduate teaching practice? If not, what are their views regarding this, particularly if it is something you are interested in developing?
- Are they involved in any primary care research activity?
- Is their contract based on general medical services (GMS) or personal medical services (PMS)? What is their performance at the QOF like?
- How much holiday do they take? What about study leave?
- Do they have a coffee room? Do they have a joint coffee break during their surgeries? This can be a really useful insight into how much they talk to one another.
- Do they have sabbaticals built into their practice agreement? How are these funded? Are there any restrictions on what you can use your sabbatical time for?
- What does the partnership agreement say about maternity rights and sick pay?
- In what circumstances can the partnership be dissolved? Is there a 'green socks' clause, where, if the majority of the partners agree, they can get rid of one individual for any reason such as they dislike his or her green socks?
- Does the partnership agreement contain references to the Mental Health Act? Some practices immediately dispel any partner who is sectioned under the Mental Health Act. While you might hope that this doesn't apply to you, does this tell you something about the practice's attitude to mental health issues?

ACTION POINT 2

Talk to your trainer and practice manager about what being a partner involves. Consider asking to see the practice accounts and partnership agreement so you can see what to look out for in the future.

Salaried

Salaried GPs are a relatively recent addition to UK general practice but they are becoming increasingly common as a means of employment. This is because prior to the introduction of the GMS contract in 2003 there was a financial incentive for practices to take on new partners, by means of the partnership allowance. This has now been incorporated into the global sum* that is paid

---

* Global sum: typically at least half of a practice's income will come from the global sum. The exact amount is calculated based on the workload from each of its patients. For example, the global sum takes into account age and gender of patients, levels of mortality and morbidity in the local area, the number of registered patients in nursing and residential homes (who have a higher workload), patient list turnover (newer patients tend to need more services than long-established ones) and a market forces factor, which reflects staff costs locally.

to practices, so it is up to the partnership whether they decide to replace any outgoing doctor with a partner or a salaried employee. How much influence you have within the practice will vary hugely, with different practices having a different ethos. You should have relative clinical freedom, at least when dealing with patients on an individual basis. Ideally you should also be involved in clinical meetings, although this can be challenging if you work part-time, because of the timings of the meetings. However, you will not be involved in business issues around employing staff or maintaining the building.

Sometimes salaried posts are used as a stepping stone to partnership, as it enables both parties to check each other out. However, if a post is advertised as 'salaried with a view', it is worth trying to get the practice to commit to a definite timescale. Otherwise, you may find yourself continually trying to impress the partners without any sense of reward.

As the name suggests, salaried roles include a regular pay packet, so you can budget for what you will take home each month. Usually this is less than you would earn as a partner in the same practice, in recognition of the fact that it carries less responsibility and also less risk. The BMA has negotiated national terms and conditions regarding GMS practices, which include study leave, sick pay and maternity rights, among other things. PMS practices are not bound by the same contractual obligations but are expected to offer employment that is 'no less favourable' than that offered by GMS practices.

It is worth remembering that as a salaried employee you are potentially vulnerable to redundancy, which, while unusual, has become a reality for some salaried GPs. When you start in the practice it is worth checking whether they are calculating your continuity of service for all your NHS employment, which they should if you have not had any career breaks, or from when you started as their practice employee. This is important, as it will make a real difference to some of your employment rights, such as maternity leave and sick pay as well as any redundancy arrangements. Also, unlike your previous NHS employment, there are no fixed pay scales for salaried GPs, although there are national guidelines, so this can vary significantly between practices.

If you are a BMA member then one of the services that they will offer you is that of contract checking, which is worth thinking about, particularly if you are going to take up a post in an unfamiliar practice. The BMA has also published a handbook for salaried GPs.[1]

You could also get a salaried position working for an alternative provider of medical services (APMS), such as Virgin Care or Harmoni, as they run some walk-in centres and out-of-hours provision. Such positions suit some individuals but it is worth checking your terms and conditions carefully, as this may well be more like those in the commercial world than the NHS, which is, generally, a good employer. It is also possible that your pay from an APMS provider may not be eligible for the NHS pension scheme, which, while it probably seems a long way off at the moment, is worth considering, as it could have a significant impact in the future.

Some practices include paying your medical indemnity as part of your salary, so you will need to consider this when comparing rates of pay. However, medical indemnity insurance is a deductible tax expense from your income so remember to take this into account when considering how much it is worth.

ACTION POINT 3

If you are a BMA member then check out the BMA publication *Focus on Salaried GPs* (available at: https://bma.org.uk/practical-support-at-work/contracts/sessional-gps/salaried-gps-handbook).

Locum

Many GP trainees start out as locums when they first qualify, as it can be a good way of finding out about how different practices work, and also getting yourself known in the local area. This can be particularly helpful if you move area after qualifying, as permanent positions are often not formally advertised but are instead signposted to likely candidates who might consider applying. So being a locum can be a good stepping stone to a permanent role, but there are also an increasing number of GPs who continue long term as locums because it suits them so well.

> My wife finished training before me and she is working as a locum. So she sees how lots of practices work, which is really interesting. I think it is probably a good way to find out if you suit a practice before taking on a permanent role.
>
> Hussein

There are three main ways in which locums are employed: (1) directly by the practice concerned, (2) via an agency or (3) via a GP locum chambers.

Approaching practices directly is probably one of the best ways to get work, although it will require a degree of organisation on your part. The first step is to identify potential practices to work in. This involves deciding how far you are prepared to travel to work. This distance will vary, depending upon whether you are in a rural or urban area but you could make an initial decision as to the ideal maximum distance and then extend this if you find that actually there will be very few opportunities for work within that area.

Having identified the area, and the practices that are within it, you then need to contact the practice managers and suggest that you are available for work. We will touch on curriculum vitaes (CVs) later in this chapter but an important thing to consider is how you would like practices to contact you. The usual method is either email or mobile phone, but whichever you choose, it is important that practices can rely on a prompt response from you, even if it is to say that you are not available on this occasion. You might also like to consider what you put in your covering letter to accompany your CV. This could include your positive attributes but it would also be sensible to include any restrictions – for example, if you can only work mornings, or can never work on Tuesdays, then say this. Although it is better to phrase it positively, such as: 'I am available to work every day, apart from Tuesdays'. If the reason that you cannot work on a particular day might make you more attractive to the practice then use it to your advantage: 'I am available every day of the week except Tuesdays, when I work as a clinical assistant at the local hospice'.

It will take some time for you to get work initially so don't panic if it is slow to filter in. It is likely that you will end up turning down work in due course. If you are offered lots of sessions in one practice that you are unfamiliar with you might like to consider accepting just one or two sessions initially so you can see how the practice functions, rather than risking finding yourself committed to something you would like to get out of. Training practices are all of a good clinical standard, as that is part of the requirements of becoming a training environment. However, this can mean that you have been cushioned from the reality of a lot of general practice – particularly, unfortunately, in an inner city environment.

You will need to ensure that you get appropriate medical indemnity cover for working as a locum, as well as registering as self-employed with Inland Revenue (see www.hmrc.gov.uk/selfemployed/register-selfemp.htm) within 3 months of starting work. You also need to think about what you would do if you were unable to work for a period of time, such as if you become unwell, as you will not be eligible for any employment benefits such as sick pay. You may have enough in savings to be able to cover your mortgage for a few months or you may consider taking out some sort of insurance policy for income protection. It is worth getting some advice from an independent financial advisor regarding this, and it would be sensible to choose someone who has experience of working with doctors. Some day release schemes have sessions covering these aspects toward the end of training; if yours doesn't, then it is worth talking to your PDs to see if one can be arranged.

You will also need to be on the performers list of wherever you intend to do the majority of your work. In April 2013, with the abolition of primary care trusts, the responsibility for holding the performers list has transferred to the NHS Commissioning Board. There is now a national performers list, which will hopefully make life easier for individuals who move geographical areas or whose work is spread across different areas. You still need to identify your local area team, which is based on your postcode, as this will have implications for your appraisal and revalidation. If you are simply continuing on as a GP after completing your training, then getting on the performers list is straightforward (www.performer.england.nhs.uk).* It is worth remembering that inclusion on the performers list is dependent upon you providing primary medical services. This means that you will not be eligible for inclusion (or retention) on the list if you stop practising as a GP or go overseas for 12 months or more.

Pay for locum work directly contracted to practices is eligible for the NHS pension scheme. Before their abolition in April 2013, primary care trusts would be responsible for the employer's contribution of the pension (on receipt of the appropriate forms). However, this has now all changed, with the employing practice now being expected to take on this cost (which is currently 14% of the pensionable amount of your fees), and being reimbursed for it via the global sum. You still have to complete the appropriate pension forms and then submit them to the appropriate authority. You will also have to include a cheque to cover both the employer and the employee pension contributions each month. If you would like more information about GP pensions then check out the NHS Business Services Authority website (www.nhsbsa.nhs.uk). The two main forms that you need are Form A, which relates to the work undertaken for a particular practice (in one calendar month), and Form B, which is a summary of all your GP locum work in that month.

Working for a locum agency may suit you if you tend to be less organised, as they effectively book the work for you and then you turn up to the practice as arranged. However, there are significant downsides to this approach. First, the fact that practices tend to pay more for agency locums than by employing individuals direct means that this tends to be the last resort for practices. So you may find yourself working in disorganised practices that are not good at planning for the absences of partners or salaried employees. Also, even though the practice pays more to the agency, that does not mean that your pay will be higher, as the agency will take a significant cut for arranging the work. Indeed, unlike when you arrange work yourself, you will not have the flexibility to decide your own pay rate.

Another thing to consider is that the locum agency often employs quite stringent terms in their contract. This usually means that if your first session with a particular practice is via an agency then they will consider themselves to have 'introduced you'. So you would not be permitted to book future work directly with that practice (even though that might be to both you and the practice's mutual benefit), at least for a number of months after initially working there.

Finally, because the contract is between you and the locum agency, rather than between you and a practice, it will not be eligible for the NHS pension scheme. In many ways it is akin to working for an APMS provider although you are still unlikely to have the employment benefits associated with being a salaried employee.

---

* To get on the Performers List in other areas of the UK please check out the information about GP registers on the GMC website at www.gmc-uk.org/doctors/registration_applications/10049.asp

GP chambers are a relatively recent innovation into the GP locum market and they can give you many of the benefits of working for a locum agency without the downsides. How it works is effectively as 'a virtual practice'. All of the members are self-employed but they use some of their earnings to employ a practice manager who co-ordinates the booking of all the work. The contract remains between the practice and the individual doctor doing the work, so it is all-eligible for the NHS pension scheme. The rate of pay is consistent among all members of the chambers but is decided between them and regularly reviewed. The chambers also serve as a learning environment where members can meet to discuss significant event audits and similar, so making preparation for revalidation easier.

The BMA has recently published a helpful handbook[2] for locum GPs.

ACTION POINT 4

- Check out BMJ Learning's information about being a successful GP locum (available at: http://learning.bmj.com/learning/module-intro/career-essentials---how-to-be-a-successful-locum-gp-.html?moduleId=10035638).

Starting out as a GP locum working peripatetically across a range of practices can initially seem rather daunting. There is paperwork to be completed but this really isn't very onerous and you will soon get used to it. Developing networks with other sessional GPs, particularly if you have moved areas, can be really helpful and it is worth exploring local sessional GP groups or joining the National Association of Sessional GPs (www.nasgp.org.uk). If paperwork really isn't your thing, there are also an increasing number of commercially available websites that will help you sort out draft invoices and pension forms and to keep track of payments.

TABLE 6.1 Comparison of different employment options

	GP principal	Salaried GP	Locum
Earning potential	Take 'drawings' from the practice, which can go up or down, but generally higher than their salaried colleagues	Generally less than GP principals or locums When comparing pay for different jobs, check what they include (e.g. does the practice pay your medical indemnity insurance?)	Variable, depending on how much you would like to work
Job security	Lifelong, once mutual assessment period is over (unless partnership breaks down or becomes insolvent, which is rare) Would be unusual to take up a partnership if you were planning to move within 5 years	Determined by the details of your contract – may be fixed term or permanent	None, although work is usually not in short supply
Influence	Complete (may not include decisions around the building if you are not a property-owning partner)	Very variable depending on practice but is, at best, likely to only include clinical aspects	None, beyond the patient whom you see in front of you
Maternity rights	Check the partnership agreement (before signing it) – 6 months is usual	Depends on details of your contract but usually up to 6 months, depending on length of service in the NHS	None except statutory rights
Sick pay	Usually participate in a locum insurance scheme as part of the practice agreement so continue to receive drawings	Depends on the details of your contract but can often be up to 6 months full pay depending on length of service in the NHS	None except statutory rights, could take out personal income protection insurance
Flexibility	Depends on whether you work full- or part-time and the partnership's view of outside interests	Can fit in well part-time with other interests	Absolutely – this is the main advantage!

HOW DO YOU FIND OUT ABOUT JOBS?

If you get the *British Medical Journal* (*BMJ*) then this will obviously be a rich source of job advertisements, provided that you make sure that you are getting the right version! Only last week one of our local GP trainers commented on how many jobs for consultant neurosurgeons there were, rather than GP jobs, and it was only then that he realised that he had been getting the wrong version for many years! However, advertising in the *BMJ* is expensive, so many practices will choose to economise and use a more informal approach, particularly for more short-term positions. Some may also advertise in the free publications such as *Pulse* or *GP* magazine.

Where jobs are advertised varies between areas; however, a good place to start is looking at the local medical committee (LMC) website and getting in touch with the local postgraduate centre, which may hold an email list through which they circulate both job opportunities and also details of educational events. If the postgraduate department is not that organised, then staying in touch with your GP training PDs or making contact with them if you move area is also useful, as practices often use them to distribute details of job vacancies.

Networking is also of key importance, as general practice jobs are often sign-posted to likely applicants rather than being formally advertised. If you are keen to get a permanent job then it is worth putting some planning into choosing where to work to get your face known. For example, if a partnership where it seems likely some individuals will retire imminently offers a long-term locum position then it may be worth considering this, as it will be a useful way of checking one another out. Whereas if you are new to an area you might like to spread your net wider and do a number of short-term locums in a variety of different practices. Joining a local locum group can also be helpful in ensuring you are aware of any potential job opportunities, as well as helping to decrease your potential professional isolation. Attending local educational events can also help in this respect, as well as giving you added benefits of maintaining your CPD. Another area to consider would be getting involved in the OOH service, particularly if you move area after finishing your training, as this can be a good way of getting to meet lots of local GPs, even if OOH is not your preferred final career option.

Finding the job that you want to apply for may take some time. Some individuals are fortunate enough to be able to obtain permanent employment as soon as they finish their GP training, but do not despair if this is not you. Being patient can pay rich dividends, provided that you use this time wisely and are proactive rather than just waiting for a job to land in your lap.*

Phrase notes
* 'land in your lap' – to be given something of value without requesting it or putting in any effort to achieve it

WHAT RESEARCH DO YOU NEED TO DO?

Once you have identified a job that you would like to consider applying for it is worth finding out as much as you can about it. Most job adverts will have a contact that you can approach for more information, such as a person specification. There may also be opportunities to undertake an informal visit. Taking advantage of these is clearly essential and can provide useful valuable information. However, it is worth remembering that this may also be the first opportunity that the practice has to get an impression of you, as well as vice versa, so think carefully about how you present yourself.

You should also seek out other ways of corroborating the information that you get from the practice. You could look at the practice website and also see if they have been rated by any patients on NHS Choices. You could also chat to your networking contacts – have any of them done any locums there, for example? Do you know any ex-GP registrars who have trained there? If so are they applying for the job? If they are not applying why is this? They may have good reason, such as moving area or wanting more or fewer hours, but it is worth finding out. If you are considering applying for a salaried post then it is certainly worth checking that you chat to one of their existing salaried employees if there are any. An outgoing salaried employee may be a particularly valuable source of information and it is always worth finding out why they are leaving.

Also remember that there is nothing to stop you asking for the person specification of a job that you would not consider applying for, particularly if it is in a geographically distant area. This might help to give you some sense of what people are looking for and help you to target your professional development to ensure that you are better prepared if a similar job came up in your local area.

WRITING YOUR CURRICULUM VITAE

Unless you get a job in your training practice then it is likely that receiving your CV, and possibly a covering letter, will be one of the first impressions that any practice has of you. So it is important to make it count and to think about how you might stand out from the crowd.

One of the first things to remember is to tailor your CV to the job on offer. If you have skills that particularly fit with those that they are looking for then make reference to these, as this demonstrates that you have read the job description. However, also think about what aspects you need to remove from your CV: you may be very proud of what you achieved in the paediatric intensive care unit but is this really relevant to a job in primary care? So while you may have a standard CV, it is likely that you will need to amend this for each application. Many individuals keep a reference CV for their own use that details all of their employment and achievements and so forth that they update regularly. This can then form the solid basis of a more tailored CV that you create for each job opportunity. It also saves you having to search repeatedly for your dates of qualification, or other key information each time.

Some basic principles are outlined here.

- Keep it concise.
- Keep it simple – don't be tempted to use fancy fonts or colours; the most usual is Times New Roman or Arial, size 12.
- Avoid long blocks of text that are hard to read.
- Include a 'career statement' on the first page – this should link to the person/job specification and show how your skills and attributes link to what they are looking for.
- Make it personal – include some personal details that describe who you are as a person, if you can link these to positive attributes so much the better (e.g. playing in the local netball team has enhanced your team-working skills).
- Include your contact details, and make sure these are up to date and accessible; try to have a professional-sounding email address – perhaps even an NHS one if you have one that you can access regularly.
- Include core information such as your GMC number and performers list registration, which the practice can then check online; if your professional name differs from that in your contact details, then take care to be accurate with this detail.
- If you are not a UK national you might like to consider including your immigration status – some individuals would argue that they do not want to draw attention to the fact that they are not British but this may well be evident already from other parts of your CV, such as your medical school or Professional and Linguistic Assessments Board (PLAB) achievements.
- Start with your most recent achievements and employment record and then work backwards – the practice is most interested in what you have done recently.
- Explain any gaps in your employment history, e.g. taking time out to look after your family – if you don't write anything then the prospective employer will be wondering what you have to hide.
- Don't include details of your schooling – does it really matter how many General Certificate of Secondary Education (or equivalent) qualifications that you got, now that you have a medical degree and MRCGP?

- Include any professional qualifications that you have achieved such as MRCGP, PLAB or diplomas.
- Include details of any relevant professional development courses that you have been on, e.g. developing teaching or leadership skills.
- Consider including details of any formal English-language qualifications that you have (such as International English Language Testing System, or IELTS) if it is obvious that English is probably not your primary language.
- Include details of any presentations or prizes, and any publications *if* they are relevant to the job in question – if you have written many publications in another clinical area, such as when pursuing an alternative career, you might consider making reference to these in broad terms rather than listing them all in detail.
- Include details of any clinical audits or other quality improvement projects that you have undertaken in practice – employers are often really interested in someone who has clearly demonstrated his or her ability to instigate and then follow through on change.
- Include details of any teaching, leadership or management skills and experience.
- Include two to three referees, including your most recent employer – if you are including their contact details ensure that they are appropriate; there is no point in including your ex-senior partner's email address if he never looks at these! You should have permission from your referees to include them. If you are going to submit your CV for multiple applications, such as short-term locum positions, then your referees may provide you with a short reference that you can use repeatedly, rather than facing numerous requests. When applying for a permanent position, it is better if your referees can target their comments to the specific job description.
- *Check it, check it and check it again!* Then get two or three objective individuals to look over it for you. Perhaps your trainer or PD might do this for you? If English is not your first language then make sure that you choose someone for whom it is to check it for you.

Remember that if the application asks for a covering letter then you need to include one, handwritten if requested (in your best handwriting!). The idea is that this and your CV should complement each other, so be careful not to just duplicate information between the two. It is likely that your covering letter will be looked at first, so this needs to be appealing enough that the readers want to find out more about you. Make sure that you address the letter accurately: getting the name of the practice manager wrong is a sure way to ensure that you are not shortlisted.

ACTION POINT 6

Write down your 'reference CV', which can then form the basis of a CV that you can adapt and tailor to each job application.

WHAT TO EXPECT AT INTERVIEW AND HOW TO PREPARE

Obviously each partnership will have a different approach as to how they interview for a position, which may be partly determined by whether it is a permanent post or not. However, there are definitely things that you can do to prepare. Remember that usually the interview process is not designed to test your clinical competence; the record of your qualifications and your referees will test this. Rather, the interview tends to focus on your character and resilience. It may also be a way in which the partners can informally test your language competency if English is not your first language.

You will have been sent the person specification and so it makes sense to start with this. An interview might well concentrate on trying to get you to provide evidence that you fulfil this. For example, if one of the criteria is to be a good team player then they may ask you to provide an example of when you have worked well in a team. Indeed for some employers, such as the civil service (who provide doctors for a variety of situations, such as civilian medical practitioners for the armed forces) this is the only type of question that they are allowed to ask. Good medical practice[3] (GMP) also forms a type of person specification, so it is worth familiarising yourself with the domains of GMP – again being able to recall examples, if asked.

> They asked me for examples of working in a team. It was really frustrating that I only thought of a good one in the car on the way home! I could have predicted that question really.
>
> Lee

Another common area that might come up in interview is what your views are in relation to some of the current hot topics within general practice. For example, at the moment you might be asked for your viewpoint on commissioning. *GP* and *Pulse* magazine are good sources of knowing what the current hot topics are, so it is worth reading these as part of your interview preparation. While you should be prepared to say what you think, and provide reasons, it is worth doing a bit of research before the interview. For example, it would be sensible to know if the senior partner is the chair of the local clinical commissioning group!

You might also be asked whether you have had any complaints and, if so, how you have dealt with this. Just like during your training, the emphasis will not be on the fact that you have had a complaint (they are an inevitable part of general practice) but on what you have learnt from it. Another common question might be whether you have had a chance to change something and, if so, what did you do and how did you approach it?

For a partnership position in particular, the interview panel may well be interested in what you can bring to the partnership beyond your clinical ability. Examples of what this might include are training aspirations, management skills or an interest in staff management. It is in this area that your prior research could pay dividends, as it may help you to identify areas in which the practice is lacking skills and expertise. However, you need to retain your integrity when discussing what additional skills you could bring. It is completely acceptable to discuss an area in which you are interested but currently lack expertise in, but you should not suggest that you are willing to take on a role that you would not enjoy or be comfortable with.

Some practices may also ask you to prepare a presentation. One local practice we know gave applicants a short summary of their current appointments system and asked individuals to think about how they would improve it. Good candidates were able to come up with realistic suggestions and to recognise that this would have implications for the wider practice staff, not just the doctors. Another practice asked individuals to bring a video of some of their consultations, as they felt this was a good way of getting a sense of the doctor's personality and whether the patients would like the doctor. Sometimes getting such evidence can be a challenge if you do not work at a regular practice, but demonstrating initiative and motivation in overcoming these potential obstacles can also provide the interviewing practice with valuable information. With the advent of revalidation there may be practices that ask you to bring your most recent MSF and/or PSQ, as every GP will have undertaken one.

Finally, it is worth remembering that an interview is in fact a two-way process and you will also have an opportunity to ask questions of your potential employers. You may of course choose not to bring up a particular issue at interview but wait until you are offered the job; however, it makes sense to have considered some of the potential sticking points in advance. In particular it is worth thinking about your negotiation skills.

Since you became a GP trainee the terms and conditions of all your posts will have been fixed, in line with NHS national arrangements. Someone has told you when you have to work and what you will be paid for doing so. General practice is different. There is no set salary, although there are certainly recommendations, and no set terms and conditions. So you need to think of these in terms of what you would consider essential and what you would consider desirable in any potential new job. If there is conflict between what you and a possible employer want, then you need to explore what the interests are that lie behind the particular position.

As with any aspect of your role, practising the skills you might need is likely to ensure that you are more prepared. Perhaps you could see if your day release course offers any sessions looking at interviews? Or what about seeing if you could swap a tutorial with another trainee where you both get a mock interview from the other's trainer? This is likely to be more effective than using your own trainer, as obviously they are already familiar to (and with) you. It is also worth talking to your trainer about what he or she might write in your reference, as these may be available to the interview panel in advance sometimes and you don't want any unwelcome surprises.

ACTION POINT 7

Ask your trainer what he or she would consider to be your strengths and areas where he or she feels you are in need of development, as this will form the basis of your reference.

WHAT ABOUT A PORTFOLIO CAREER?

One of the huge advantages of general practice is the variety of potential career options it can offer. We have touched on the principles of getting your core clinical post sorted but there is endless variety in what is available beyond this. Common examples of areas that you might like to consider exploring are outlined here.

- **Medical education**: this can range from one-to-one teaching at undergraduate to postgraduate level, such as becoming a medical student tutor, Foundation programme CS or GP trainer, to ad hoc group teaching sessions to ongoing commitment, such as a GP training PD, or university lecturer.
- **GP with a special interest**: you could develop a community-based programme such as echocardiography (perhaps drawing on any prior experience you may have had) or become involved in secondary care as a clinical assistant or staff grade.
- **Medical politics**: you could get involved in your LMC or get yourself elected to one of the BMA or RCGP committees.
- **Medical journalism**: you could write for one of the GP magazines, or the *British Journal of General Practice* or *BMJ*, or try and branch out and write for a secular magazine.
- **Forensic medicine**: you could develop skills as a police surgeon, either across the whole breadth of the criminal system or just undertaking forensic examinations following sexual assaults.
- **Research**: this could be at a practice level, providing patients as clinical material for existing research studies, or you could develop links with your local department of academic primary care.
- **Humanitarian work abroad**: you could get involved in short-term overseas

work, either as a clinician providing direct patient care or otherwise sharing your expertise and helping to develop the local healthcare provision.

- **Appraisal**: you could become an appraiser and undertake regular GP appraisals of your peers.
- **Medico-legal work**: this could range from doing insurance assessments for people to sitting on tribunal panels for individuals contesting their benefits assessment.
- **Occupational medicine**: this might include features such as doing medicals for the local bus company, or individuals wanting pilot licences.
- **Private work**: this could be health assessments for Bupa or similar, or working in a cosmetic clinic.

These are just some of the examples on offer. We are sure you can think of more – and that is without thinking beyond medicine! Finding out about opportunities is often slightly hit-and-miss. It is worth talking to someone involved in your area of interest to find out how he or she got involved and also to express

TABLE 6.2 A possible working week for a portfolio GP (a typical week for me (MF) at the end of 2013)

Monday	Tuesday	Wednesday	Thursday	Friday	Weekend
Education learning set for international graduates	GP day release course (as PD)	GP locum	Writing this book	Volunteer doctor for canal boat, taking groups of disabled people	Catching up with paperwork – sorting out invoices for work On call for hospice (from home)
GP locum	GP day release course then trainers group	Lunch – appraiser steering group meeting Then GP locum	Own GP appraisal	Appraisal	Lunch with family Doctor's session for Winston's Wish (local charity for bereaved children) explaining the medicine behind the death of their parent or sibling
Writing article for *Pulse* Teaching English as a foreign language lesson (in preparation for humanitarian work)	Telephone discussion about book proposal with fellow author	On call for local hospice overnight (based at home)	GP study group with pudding!	Planning meeting regarding aid work abroad	Theatre – to see if it would be relevant for teaching? (and also very enjoyable!)

your interest so that he or she will know that you exist. For example, an individual interested in medical education might well talk to his or her local PDs and offer to teach some sessions to the group. That way if a job opportunity became available then the existing team would be likely to signpost it to you and you would be in a good position to apply.

However, remember that two part-time jobs usually add up to more than one full-time position! Also, portfolio GPs tend to be lower earners than their GP partner colleagues, although this is not always the case. The way in which you are paid may also change and will probably include some areas where you are paid for your results, such as the submission of an article, rather than for the time taken to complete the piece of work. You also need to make sure that you carve out time for yourself, such as holidays, as otherwise you may find yourself never being in a position to take a proper break.

ACTION POINT 8

Think about what areas, if any, interest you outside core general practice. Is this something you would like to explore further? How might you go about that?

WHAT IF YOU DIDN'T MAKE IT?

It took me some time to come to terms with what had happened. At first it just seemed so unreal. But it gradually sank in. It was great to be able to do some locums in the A&E department where I had been a GP trainee. It helped my pride that they were willing, indeed keen, to have me back and it enabled me to feed my family.

As for the longer term, well I'm working on that.

Daniel

Unfortunately, some of you reading this book may not successfully complete your GP training – for example, after multiple exam failures. So what about you? Obviously it makes sense to explore any of the appeal opportunities available to you, but once these have been exhausted you need to think about what to do next. Well, first of all don't rush into any long-term decisions, and second, don't panic! There are still plenty of job opportunities available to you, even if the door to becoming a UK GP has been shut.

Initially you will probably be in the first stages of a grief reaction, with anger and denial of the reality of what has happened. Recognising this, and accepting that it is an understandable response to events, is part of moving on. For you will move on, to the acceptance part of the grief reaction.

When you are ready, take a step back and think about the values that are important to you. You are still the same individual you were before this setback, with the same values and priorities. So what makes you tick?* Take advantage of any help that is on offer in helping to work these issues through. Most deaneries have some form of professional development unit that offers career guidance. Usually these will have been signposted to you when it looked possible that you might end up being released from training but, if not, ask your PDs about what is available locally. It is much easier to work through these difficult issues with some external support.

The next thing to do is to think about why it is that you didn't make it. This is the time to be honest with yourself, and give others permission to be honest too. Think about who you trust to be able to give you this feedback. Who knows your strengths and your weaknesses? Who can you rely on to tell you things that you may not want to hear?

However, you need to be in the right place emotionally to be able to achieve this. If you are still railing at the perceived unfairness of your current predicament, then you need more time. However, if you have managed to accept the reality of your situation, then this can be a crucial stage in helping you decide what to do next, and how to avoid facing similar issues in the future. So it would be great to make sure that you have some people in your life who will support you unreservedly, such as family and friends, and others who have permission to discuss honestly with you the options available, such as your ES and PD.

Things you might like to consider are outlined here.

- Are you suited to the independent nature of GP practice or are you better as part of a larger clinical team?
- Was general practice your first choice of specialty? If not, what was? Why didn't you pursue that option? Is it something you can revisit?
- If you have previously pursued another specialty, what happened? If you didn't succeed there either, then are there any recurring themes that you need to try and address?
- Can you be patient centred in the way that UK general practice demands? Or do you always find yourself reverting to a doctor-centred approach?
- What did you enjoy about general practice? What did you find more of a challenge?
- Were there any jobs that you particularly enjoyed as part of your GP training? What was it about them that attracted you?
- Being completely honest, are your English-language skills up to the job? If not, how could you improve them? Is this a realistic aspiration?
- Why did you come to the UK? Is this your home or could you consider moving back to your country of origin?

Phrase notes

* 'makes you tick' – something that motivates you or encourages you to behave in a particular way

- Why did you go into medicine originally? Was it your dream or that of your family? Do you still enjoy medicine?
- What are your personal and family circumstances? Can you afford to take some time out or do you need to be earning a good salary in order to pay off debts?

> My father wanted me to study medicine because he was thinking of all the good I could offer mankind. Be altruistic, ethical, moral, 'to save the world'. And foolish me I listened …
>   How many times have I regretted listening?
>
> Katya

Deciding what to do next will be very different for every individual. Just like deciding what your dream practice would look like, there is no right or wrong answer, just the right answer *for you*. You need to go back to the first principles of your underlying values and, only when you have established what these are, start to overlay them with the practicalities that you need to consider. You also need to get over any sense of humiliation that you may feel and take advantage of all the help that is on offer to you. Remember that qualifying as a doctor and then being accepted onto a UK GP training scheme are real achievements that would be beyond the reach of many. Try to keep your current predicament in perspective – worse things happen at sea.[*]

Some people will end up continuing to explore a different branch of medicine, whereas others may decide that medicine is not for them. The important thing, whatever you decide, is to try to set aside your regret at what might have been and start living the life you now want. Engaging with a life coach, or critical friend, may be helpful at this time of enormous transition. There are numerous publications and websites that can help you at this point in time. Examples might include Medical Forum (http://medicalforum.com) or Medical Success (http://medicalsuccess.net) or books such as those by Susan Kersley.[4,5]

ACTION POINT 9

Who can you identify as being a possible 'critical friend', helping you to honestly identify both your strengths and your areas for development?

Phrase notes
[*] 'worse things happen at sea' – a way of telling someone not to worry so much about his or her problems

WHAT IF YOU DECIDE IT IS NOT FOR YOU?

It is also possible that you may have successfully completed your GP training but reached the conclusion that general practice is not for you. If that is how you are feeling, then you need to take a similar approach to those who didn't make it and try to work out what your core values are. This may help you to determine whether it is the whole of general practice that doesn't suit you or whether you are simply in the wrong practice. For the world of general practice is so varied that it may well be that changing practice, or exploring an outside interest to complement your clinical work, will have a dramatic effect on your professional satisfaction.

> By the time I got to the end I hated my job. I think that all the stress of exams had affected me. So I went on holiday with my wife and we thought about what to do. We even considered going back home to Iraq but that wasn't right for our family. So I just got on with finding a job. And now I enjoy it again as the practice is so different from my training one. My patients like me, and I like them.
>
> Jamail

Again it is worth seeking outside input[4] to help you explore some of these issues. Your previous ES would be a good place to start, as he or she has developed some good insights into what makes you tick. There may also be a mentoring scheme run locally and designed specifically for newly qualified GPs; these are often accessed via the deanery or your local RCGP faculty. Sometimes the career support services offered by deaneries to their trainees are also available to qualified practitioners (although they may not remain free of charge) so again these are worth investigating.

There may also be some advantages in taking some time out to explore your options. If you think another branch of medicine might suit you better, then why not see if you can get some experience in that specialty to see how it really is. You can always return to general practice at a later date and your experience of GP training will not be wasted. It is worth knowing, however, that if you are out of practice for 2 years then you will probably need to undergo some retraining, which may well be at your own expense. So if you are still unsure it may be worth keeping your options open by at least doing some occasional GP locum sessions.

> I was very happy and over the moon when I achieved my goals and my dreams came true of being an obstetrician with the higher exams I needed for Iraq, and all the Arabic countries. Then we had to face the invasion of the Americans, which had a huge impact on all our lives. I was without a job for many months during and after the invasion.
>
> I didn't want to change and now I have a decision to make. Do I go back to obstetrics? Can I face more years of training? What about all the work I have out into general practice – will that be wasted too?
>
> Sana'a

CONTINUING YOUR PROFESSIONAL DEVELOPMENT

Getting your dream job is obviously just one of the stages in your career. You will also have to continue to maintain your professional development, particularly now that revalidation has been introduced. Hopefully some of the strategies of adult learning that you developed during your GP training will help with this, but it is worth also thinking about what other methods you could use.

APPRAISAL AND REVALIDATION

You will probably have effortlessly sailed through* your first cycle of revalidation without noticing it, as it occurs at 5 years after registration or at gaining your CCT, whichever comes sooner. Requirements such as MSF and a PSQ will have been easy to achieve, as they are part of the formal components of WPBA. However, next time they may not be so straightforward, so it is worth thinking about what you will need to do to prepare.

Enhanced GP appraisal, by one of your peers, is the cornerstone of revalidation[6] and you will need to participate in this on an annual basis. Your final Educational Supervisor's Report will count as your first appraisal but, particularly given that this occurs some time before the actual end of training, it is worth thinking about whether you could also organise an NHS style appraisal. It may be that your trainer could undertake this for you but it would be worth considering getting someone else in the practice to do it, especially if you are fortunate enough to have contact with an appraiser. This will then enable you to develop a personal development plan for your first year of independent practice. You can then reflect back on it at your first formal appraisal, the following year. Having to crystallise your thinking and your plans in this way, when there is no one telling you what you *have* to do, can be really useful. It can even help you when trying to identify what your priorities might be in finding a permanent job.

> I was nervous about it but my first NHS appraisal was great. It helped me to step back and think about what to do next. I had been concentrating so much on the exams that I had forgotten what I wanted to do.
>
> Ebrahim

What you will need to bring to your NHS appraisal is supporting information in the following categories.
- **General information**: providing the context of everything you do in all aspects of your work – this would include any extra roles that you might

---

Phrase notes
* 'sailed through' – to achieve something easily with little apparent effort

have, such as being involved in GP education or as a clinical assistant in a hospital clinic, for example.

- **Keeping up to date**: maintaining and enhancing the quality of your professional work.
- **Review of your practice**: your own evaluation of the quality of your professional work.
- **Feedback on your practice**: how others view the quality of your professional work.

How you demonstrate this is largely up to you and there are a variety of portfolios available to help you keep records of your learning. Some of these, such as the RCGP one, will even highlight to you what aspects may be missing for this cycle of revalidation, as some items are only needed once every 5 years.

Every year you will be expected to provide a record of your learning activities and the recommended minimum is 50 learning credits. Just like during your GP training, you will get more credit for learning that has had a more significant impact on your practice. For example, learning about a new drug interaction highlighted by the Medicines and Healthcare Products Regulatory Agency will have greater significance if you then share your learning with your colleagues and undertake an audit of patients who have been prescribed the relevant drugs. Doing such an audit would also count as a quality improvement activity which is something you will be encouraged to do each year. Other examples of quality improvement activities might include a case review, or the implementation of a change in the practice, such as adapting the appointments system. You will also be expected to reflect on any significant events that have occurred during your practice, as well as to reflect on any complaints that you may have been involved in.

Once in every revalidation cycle (i.e. every 5 years) you will be expected to get formal feedback from your colleagues and your patients. This can sometimes present a practical challenge, particularly if you do not have a regular practice base. So it is worth keeping them in mind and seizing any opportunities that might present themselves, such as when doing a long-term maternity locum, rather than waiting until the last minute. There are a variety of tools available to help you do this. Some of them are free of charge, whereas others charge a fee for their service but in exchange often take away a lot of the administrative hassle that may otherwise accompany it.

As you can probably tell this should not really be too much of an ordeal for you. You are used to recording your learning and getting feedback from patients and colleagues as part of your progression through WPBA. It may be more of a challenge for your more senior counterparts for whom such assessments are a new endeavour. Ideally, each year your appraisal should look at whether you are on track for successful revalidation or if there are particular areas that you need to focus on.

ACTION POINT 10

Find a GP appraiser who might be prepared to undertake an NHS style appraisal with you as you come to the end of your training.

MAINTAINING YOUR LEARNING

There are many ways that you can maintain your learning to ensure that you remain on track for revalidation. You can certainly continue to use strategies that worked for you in training, such as using patients as a stimulus for learning. If you regularly use resources such as GPnotebook during consultations, it is worth making sure that you log into it at the start of each surgery, as it will then automatically track your learning, which you can then provide as evidence at your appraisal without any further effort. You can also continue to participate in online learning modules, many of which will also be automatically tracked if you log into the relevant websites.

Many people, however, value some group learning, as it helps to maintain their enthusiasm. Sometimes small groups from your vocational training scheme continue following completion of training, particularly given that many people stay in the same geographical area. Sometimes like-minded individuals form groups – for example, locum groups are relatively common – but we also know of groups of mums of young children who meet together for learning activities. The RCGP has also developed the First Five initiative of groups, designed specifically for individuals who are, as the name suggests, within 5 years of completing their training. These can be a particularly useful resource to tap into if you move area on completing your training, as they will enable you to develop networks with a new group of colleagues.

Another source of group learning can be a local educational trust. These are often facilitated via the postgraduate education centres and usually involve you signing up for a year. Having signed up you can then attend as many local events as you like, which is usually really good value for money, as well as providing useful networking opportunities. There may also be reciprocal arrangements with neighbouring educational trusts whereby you can also attend their events free, or at a reduced cost.

Then there are the commercially available courses, ranging from the broad-brush courses reviewing the latest evidence base to masterclasses concentrating on a particular clinical area. Your medical indemnity organisation may also provide some interesting courses, which are often free of charge to members.

ACTION POINT 11

Talk to some of your colleagues at the day release course. Would they be interested in continuing to form a study group for the future?

MENTORING

As already mentioned, mentoring can also be a really helpful tool in continuing your professional development. The one-to-one relationship that you will have had with your trainer during your final year is often very intense, particularly if you have shared challenges such as exam failures together. So when you move out into independent practice the loss of this supportive relationship can lead to a real sense of professional isolation, particularly if you do not move immediately into a permanent position. Building new relationships and professional support takes time and engaging in a mentoring scheme can really help in this regard. So it is worth seeking out what might be available in your local area. If there is no scheme it is worth asking your local RCGP faculty as to whether one could be designed. Or you could explore persuading one of your colleagues from your vocational training scheme if they would consider developing a co-mentoring relationship with you, where you take it in turns to mentor each other.

The point of developing a mentoring relationship is in enabling you to develop and generate your own solutions rather than the mentor aiming to be an expert and provide solutions, which may or may not be appropriate for you. Using a model to guide the mentoring may facilitate this, although, as with any model, being flexible in how you apply it is essential. Two common models that are used in a healthcare setting are the GROW model[7] and Egan's Skilled Helper[8] model.

The GROW model is:
- Goals – what do you want?
- Reality – what is happening now?
- Options – what could you do now?
- Will – what will you do now?

Egan's Skilled Helper model is:
- What is going on (the present)?
- What solutions make sense for me (the future)?
- How do I get what I need or want (linking the present and the future)?

If you are going to take on the role of co-mentoring one of your colleagues, it would make sense to read some more about mentoring. A good place to start would be with the book *Coaching and Mentoring at Work*.[9] You could even make that one of your objectives on your first PDP!

> Finding a mentor was my salvation. She helped me to see that there was more to general practice than my current practice. She gave me the confidence to resign, even though I didn't have another job to go to. And I have never looked back. Now I complement my GP work with palliative care at the local hospice and I love it.
>
> Simone

LOOKING FORWARD

This chapter has looked at what you might explore next after completing your GP training. Obviously it can only touch on the options available for you but hopefully it has given you some food for thought. Navigating the MRCGP exam is literally the first step in years of a fulfilling career in general practice. Whether you take our approach of the portfolio career or that of the senior partner's who spent more than 35 years in the same community, the world really is your oyster. Being a medic, and in particular, a GP, is a passport to opportunity.

> I am eagerly waiting to serve my community as an independent, good GP.
>
> Marcus

> I am now a practising GP and I am enjoying it. It is one of the best decisions I have made with regard to my career.
>
> Gloria

REFERENCES

1. British Medical Association (BMA). *Salaried GP Handbook*. London: BMA, 2010. Available at: https://bma.org.uk/practical-support-at-work/contracts/sessional-gps/salaried-gps-handbook (accessed 2 May 2013).
2. British Medical Association (BMA). *Locum GP Handbook*. London: BMA; 2012. Available at: https://bma.org.uk/practical-support-at-work/contracts/sessional-gps/locum-gp-handbook (accessed 2 May 2013).
3. General Medical Council (GMC). *Good Medical Practice*. London: GMC; 2013. Available at: www.gmc-uk.org/guidance/good_medical_practice.asp (accessed 2 May 2013).
4. Kersley SE. *Life After Medicine*. Oxford: Radcliffe Publishing; 2010.
5. Kersley SE. *Prescription for Change: for doctors who want a life*. Oxford: Radcliffe Publishing; 2006.

6. General Medical Council (GMC). *My Revalidation*. London: GMC; 2012. Available at: www.gmc-uk.org/doctors/revalidation/12382.asp (accessed 2 May 2013).

7. Whitmore J. *Coaching for Performance: GROWing people, performance and purpose*. 3rd ed. London: Nicholas Brealey; 2002.

8. Egan G. *The Skilled Helper*. 7th ed. Belmont, CA: Thomson Books/Cole; 2002.

9. Connor M, Pokora J. *Coaching and Mentoring at Work: developing effective practice*. Maidenhead: Open University Press; 2007.

List of abbreviations

A&E	accident and emergency
AiT	Associate in Training
AKT	Applied Knowledge Test (part of the MRCGP exam)
ALS	advanced life support
APMS	alternative provider of medical services
ARCP	annual review of competence of progression
BLS	basic life support
BMA	British Medical Association
BMJ	*British Medical Journal*
CbD	case-based discussion
CCT	certificate of completion of training
COT	consultation observation tool (part of WBPA in GP posts)
CPD	continuing professional development
CS	clinical supervisor
CSA	Clinical Skills Assessment (part of the MRCGP exam)
CSR	Clinical Supervisor's Report
CV	curriculum vitae
DOPS	Direct Observation of Procedural Skills
ES	educational supervisor
EQ	emotional intelligence
EWTD	European Working Time Directive
GMC	General Medical Council
GMP	good medical practice
GMS	General Medical Services
GP	general practitioner
GPStR	general practice specialty registrar
IELTS	International English Language Testing System
IMG	international medical graduate (someone who qualified outside the UK)
InnovAiT	RCGP journal aimed at AiTs

LETB	local education and training board
LMC	local medical committee
Mini-CEX	Mini Clinical Evaluation Exercise (part of WPBA in hospital posts)
MRCGP	Membership of the Royal College of General Practitioners
MSF	multi-source feedback (part of WPBA)
NHS	National Health Service
NICE	National Institute for Health and Care Excellence
OMG	overseas medical graduate
OOH	out of hours
PACES	Membership of the Royal College of Physicians Part 2 Clinical Examination
PD	programme director
PDP	personal development plan
PLAB	Professional and Linguistic Assessments Board
PMS	personal medical services
PSQ	Patient Satisfaction Questionnaire (part of WPBA)
QOF	Quality and Outcomes Framework
RCGP	Royal College of General Practitioners
SEA	significant event analysis
St1	specialty training year 1
St2	specialty training year 2
St3	specialty training year 3
UK	United Kingdom
WPBA	workplace-based assessment (part of the MRCGP exam)

Commonly used idioms and colloquialisms

This is not intended to be an exhaustive list and we would encourage you to ask patients to explain if they use an expression that you do not understand.

Expression	Meaning
absent-minded	forgetful
all done in	exhausted
at my wits' end	unable to do any more or carry on
at the end of my tether	unable to do any more or carry on
away with the fairies	confused
balls	testicles
befuddled	confused
bit icky	nauseous
bit on the side	sexual partner who is not your significant other
blew a fuse/blew a gasket	angry
boobies	breasts
buggered	tired
bunged up	constipated
burning up	feverish
butterflies in my stomach	anxious
cack-handed	awkward/clumsy (occasionally means left-handed)
can't get it up	can't get an erection
carked it	died
cheesed off	upset/cross

Expression	Meaning
chundering	vomiting
close shave	saved from serious injury/death
come on	started my menses/period
couch potato	lazy, spending lots of time on the sofa
done like the dog's dinner	tired
down below	perineum, usually vulval/vaginal area
down in the dumps	depressed
driving me barmy	making me very angry or impatient
dropped off	fell asleep
end it all	commit suicide
fall off the wagon	to relapse, e.g. in alcoholism
fallen off his perch	died
fanny	vagina
feeling a bit iffy	feeling unwell
feeling woozy	dizzy or light-headed
fizzy/pins and needles	paraesthesiae
frog in my throat	hoarse/croaky voice
front bottom	vagina
gammy leg	painful leg
gave me a blank look	didn't understand
get it off my chest	tell someone else about what is worrying you
gippy tummy	diarrhoea
go cold turkey	to give up something you are dependent on without help, e.g. alcoholic who stops drinking
go doolally	confused or crazy
gone to heaven	died
got a bun in the oven	pregnant
got a dicky ticker	got a heart condition, e.g. angina
got her period	is menstruating
got Niagara Falls	is menstruating heavily
got the trots	diarrhoea
grab a pew	take a seat
gullet	oesophagus
gut rot	abdominal pain, often indigestion
had a fit	shocked

Expression	Meaning
head over heels	overjoyed
heartburn	indigestion
her indoors	wife/partner
high as a kite	intoxicated or overexcited
in cloud cuckoo land	confused
in hot water	in trouble
jerk off/wank	masturbate
keep nodding off	falling asleep
keep your chin up	think positive/be optimistic
keep your fingers crossed	hope for the best outcome
kicked the bucket	died
knackered	exhausted
knocked up	pregnant
laid off	to lose your job
leave no stone unturned	to try everything
long and short of it	main point
looking green around the gills	looking unwell or nauseous
lugholes	ears
make a mess	bowels open, particularly in nappy wearing children
manky	infected
minny	vagina
monthlies	menstrual period
monthly curse	menstrual period
my belly thinks me throat's cut	hungry
my old ticker	my heart
not on top form	feeling unwell
number 1 and number 2	passing urine (number 1) and opening bowels (number 2)
off colour	feeling unwell
off his head	confused or intoxicated
off his rocker	crazy
on cloud nine	overjoyed
on the dole	unemployed
once in a blue moon	rarely
other half	partner or wife/husband
out like a light	to go to sleep easily

Expression	Meaning
out of sorts	feeling unwell
over the moon	delighted
pack it in	give something up, e.g. smoking
parched	thirsty
passed away	died
peaky	non-specifically unwell
pie in the sky	unrealistic
pixelated	tired
popped her clogs	died
privates/private parts	genitalia
pull a fast one	to lie or pretend
pull a sickie	take a day off as sick leave when not actually unwell
pull the wool over someone's eyes	to hide the truth
pulling your leg	having a joke
put your head in the sand	ignore something in the hope it will go away
queasy	nauseous
roof's fallen in	everything has gone wrong
sandwich short of a picnic	stupid
scored an own goal	made it worse for themselves
sent him to Coventry	not talking to him
shattered	tired
she's a worrywart	someone who is always anxious
significant other	someone with whom you are in a long-term, often intimate, relationship
sloshed/tipsy/hammered/pissed	had too much alcohol to drink
snowed under	having too much to do
sofa surfer	homeless person who rotates staying with different friends
spend a penny	go to the toilet to pass urine
swinging the lead	to avoid going to work, malingering
take a duvet day	take a day off as sick leave when not actually unwell
take a leaf out of your book	follow your example
take an ostrich approach	ignore something in the hope it will go away
technicolour yawning	vomiting
the runs	diarrhoea
the snip	vasectomy

Expression	Meaning
throwing up	vomiting
time of the month	when your period/menses are due
tingling	paraesthesiae
tits	breasts
trouble and strife	wife
tummy ache	abdominal pain
turning on the waterworks	crying
twisted my arm	to be persuaded (e.g. 'my wife twisted my arm so I came along')
up the duff	pregnant
wacky backy	cannabis
water sample	urine specimen
waterworks	urinary system
wearing me down	feeling under pressure
wedding tackle	male genitalia
wet behind the ears	young or inexperienced
wet me knickers	incontinent of urine
willy	penis
windpipe	trachea

Index

Entries in **bold** refer to figures and tables.

CPD with Radcliffe

You can now use a selection of our books to achieve CPD (Continuing Professional Development) points through directed reading.

We provide a free online form and downloadable certificate for your appraisal portfolio. Look for the CPD logo and register with us at: www.radcliffehealth.com/cpd

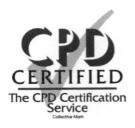